Success Is What You Leave Behind

T0383356

Success Is What You Leave Behind

Fostering Leadership and Innovation

Cato T. Laurencin, MD, PhD

University Professor,
Albert and Wilda Van Dusen Distinguished Endowed
Chair Professor of Orthopaedic Surgery,
Professor of Chemical and Biomolecular Engineering,
Professor of Materials Science and Engineering,
Professor of Biomedical Engineering,
The University of Connecticut, Storrs, CT, United States

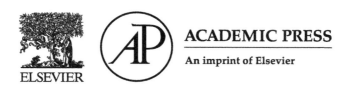

ELSEVIER

ACADEMIC PRESS

An imprint of Elsevier

Library of Congress Cataloging-in-Publication Data
A catalog record for this book is available from the Library of Congress

British Library Cataloguing-in-Publication Data
A catalogue record for this book is available from the British Library

ISBN: 978-0-12-417224-1

For information on all Academic Press publications visit our
website at https://www.elsevier.com/books-and-journals

Publisher: Mica Haley
Acquisitions Editor: Michelle Fisher
Editorial Project Manager: Pat Gonzalez
Production Project Manager: Punithavathy Govindaradjane
Cover Designer: Mark Rogers

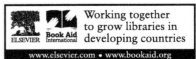

Typeset by TNQ Technologies

To my dear wife Cynthia and my wonderful children. You have all my love.

To Laura Simmons, Diane Sullivan, and Susan Fitzgerald, for your goodness, sensitivity, and kindness.

To Sherman Feir for being a good friend and truly good person.

And to my cousin Lisa Laurencin for being phenomenal.

Contents

About the Author

Cato T. Laurencin, MD, PhD, is the University Professor and Albert and Wilda Van Dusen Distinguished Endowed Professor of Orthopaedic Surgery at the University of Connecticut. In receiving the 2021 Spingarn Medal given for the "highest or noblest achievement by a living African American during the preceding year or years in any honorable field," the NAACP stated "His exceptional career has made him the foremost engineer—physician—scientist in the world. His breakthrough achievements have resulted in transformative advances in improving human life."

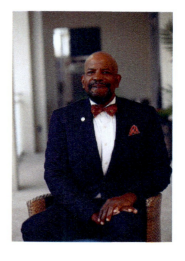

Dr. Laurencin is the first surgeon in history elected to all four National Academies: the National Academy of Sciences, the National Academy of Medicine, the National Academy of Engineering, and the National Academy of Inventors. He is the founder of the field of regenerative engineering and received the National Medal of Technology and Innovation from President Barack Obama in ceremonies at the White House, the nation's highest honor for technological achievement.

Dr. Laurencin's expertise encompasses broad areas of engineering, medicine, and science. In engineering, he received the Simon Ramo Founder's Award, the oldest/highest award of the National Academy of Engineering, In medicine, he received the Walsh McDermott Medal, one of the oldest/highest awards of the National Academy of Medicine. In science, he received the Philip Hauge Abelson Prize from the American Association for the Advancement of Science, given for "signal contributions to the advancement of science in the United States."

Dr. Laurencin is internationally renowned in engineering, medicine, and science. In engineering, he is a fellow of the Royal Academy of Engineering, a fellow of the Indian National Academy of Engineering, and an academician of the Chinese Academy of Engineering. In medicine, he received the UNESCO Equatorial Guinea International Prize for Research in the Life Sciences.

In science, he is a fellow of both the National Academy of Sciences, India and the African Academy of Sciences.

Dr. Laurencin earned his BSE in chemical engineering from Princeton University; his MD, *Magna Cum Laude*, from the Harvard Medical School; and his PhD in biochemical engineering/biotechnology from the Massachusetts Institute of Technology.

Foreword by Garth Graham, MD, MPH, FACP, FACC

Many years ago, when I was deputy assistant secretary for Minority Health at the United States Department of Health and Human Services, I attended an interesting meeting. I walked into the ballroom where I was next up to speak and observed the man at the podium commanding the room as he spoke about what we needed to do as a country to tackle the challenges of improving health for the poor and underserved and those who needed our help the most. As I saw this man speak, his grip on the room was driven not by esoteric points on science and medicine but by real-world descriptions of how we could use the tools of science and medicine to improve the lives of individuals in the community. That is where I first got introduced to the preeminent physician scientist of our generation… Dr. Cato Laurencin.

Dr. Laurencin's name means a lot to different people. As an orthopedic surgeon, his groundbreaking work in leading the treatment of shoulder and knee disease has led to him receiving the highest honors from his surgical colleagues. As an engineer, his work in musculoskeletal tissue regeneration has revolutionized the field leading to him being honored by none other than a sitting President of the United States for his technological achievements. But the essence of his work that has moved me the most are his efforts in tackling health injustices and pushing the country to achieve health equity. That's what he pushed that audience in that ballroom to do almost 20 years ago, and that's what he has pushed this nation to do over the course of his career.

This is embodied in the words, thoughts, and inspiration of this book. His life experiences, leadership, and accomplishments are an inspiration to the next generation of leaders. Over the past couple decades, I have gotten to know Dr. Laurencin as he has mentored me and many others like me through various life decisions. He is amazingly down to earth, despite his track record of achievements. He works tirelessly behind the scenes to push us to achieve things we only dreamed of, yet he does it in a discreet compassionate way shunning the limelight and the accolades. His words of wisdom have helped guide my life, and as captured in this book, it can help others who are similarly interested in leadership, impact, and change. Great leaders leave footprints in their tracks that show us the way, if success is what you leave behind, this book is a step-by-step road map to help guide us on the path to not just an impactful career but ultimately a meaningful life.

Success Is What You Leave Behind. https://doi.org/10.1016/B978-0-12-417224-1.00006-7

Preface

The late, Nobel-Prize winning author, Toni Morrison often suggested to those who wanted to know how she decided to write the books she has written. She advises us to write the books you want to read. When I was a young man on the journey, it would have been helpful to have a voice in my ear, guiding me. This is what I set out to do with this book. While it details my successes, I wanted to share the story of the lefts, rights, and pivots of how I got here. It is great to read about someone who has been able to innovate, but it is so important to motivate by sharing some of the blueprint of how it happens and how to balance work, family, and a life of service.

This book, *Success Is What You Leave Behind*, has been in the making for decades. It reflects my lived experience as a child growing up in North Philadelphia, becoming a physician, orthopedic surgeon, engineer, and scientist, and beyond. Each opportunity and challenge has brought me to this point.

Success Is What You Leave Behind is written from the perspective of one who has committed his career to building and refining solutions that will improve the quality of life for people now and in the future, and one who has dedicated himself to. It details how I and my team created a new field in science, regenerative engineering, and how we got here. This is significant and brought me accolades and awards, as well as funding to continue my work. But any scientist or researcher of note will tell you there is so much more that goes into success than the external praise.

No successful person, no matter what their profession, gets here in a vacuum. We have mentors, sponsors, and guides along the way. And I am proud to introduce you to some of these invaluable relationships.

I wrote this book to encourage and inspire those who are making decisions about their own careers now and in the future. Every time I give a speech, or have the opportunity to talk with students, I am well aware that they are looking to me to get some insights into how they can shape a sustainable and successful career.

And if they had never seen an orthopedic surgeon who is also an engineer, who has melded both of those things into science and research, this book shows that it can happen. But I also hope that it encourages the reader to not just reach for the stars but also strive to give back every step of the way.

It is my hope that the reader will read this book with themselves and what is possible in their lives, in mind.

Chapter 1

Regenerative Engineering, Convergence, and Building a New Field

The principles in medicine, engineering, and science, as well as the values and insights that I have learned along the way have helped shape my life. Many of these lessons I learned the hard way, starting when I was a kid in the Black inner-city neighborhood of North Philadelphia.

When I completed college, I went on to medical school at the Harvard Medical School in Boston, and partway through I decided to revisit my scientific and engineering routes. I met Robert Langer, who was a young assistant professor at that time and decided to join his laboratory. I subsequently took on a combined MD–PhD program combining work at Harvard with work at MIT. This program was unusual, and I realized that to do a comprehensive job on both would take a long, long time.

With the support and help of Noreen Koller, who was a fantastic registrar at Harvard, I was allowed to move back and forth for my training, so I would do clinical rotations and then I would do work in the laboratory. This enabled me to complete my MD and PhD combined in seven years, which really helped me on my journey because I became very, very used to working in both the clinical and research realms. I then began a residency in orthopaedic surgery and opened my laboratory at MIT.

Since then, I have been working in both areas; a common theme in all my research has been combining the principles of material science and engineering with physics and clinical medicine to allow us to be able to create new information and new science.

Those lessons were priceless, and yes, I am still learning them. The pursuit of excellence in your work, or in your life are never settled matters. The period at the end of the lesson becomes a comma, because if we do it right, we gain additional insights along the and keep asking, "What's next, and how can I do it better?" What makes the difference is how you manage the quest. These are, I think, some of the main rules of the road. In this case, a winding road that led me to working to build a new field within regenerative medicine. However, let me tell you about how I got here.

Success Is What You Leave Behind. https://doi.org/10.1016/B978-0-12-417224-1.00001-8

The regeneration of human limbs has been a dream of the medical and scientific communities for years. Piecing all of the elements together is like working on a puzzle. I see it as one of the important steps in 21st-century medical advances. In addition, it has become the core of my life's work. When people who do not know me ask what I do for a living, it takes my mind back to that kid from Philly. I was always interested in medicine but did not think that my answer would one day be, "I am a chemical engineer, medical scientist, and orthopaedic surgeon." All that and a pioneer in my field and as a Black man in this work, I am often seen as a bit of a unicorn. The truth is I worked hard to be in this space, and I stand here at the grace who came before me, and for those who need to see me and know that this is possible for them, too.

Heading Into Unknown Territory—Creating Something New

Medical scientists have already made great progress toward rebuilding body parts from patients' own cells. While it might seem to be the stuff of science fiction to the general public, therapies exist right now that utilize bio-engineered repairs to urethras, bladders, tracheas, and other organs. Scientists are even pursuing the far more complicated goal of creating kidneys, livers, and hearts—all starting with the patient's own harvested cells.

The science of regenerating body elements is well out of its infancy. Today, blood banks allow parents to save the placental and umbilical cord blood of their newborns, replete with stem cells that can be trained to transform themselves into any type of bodily cell. Stem cells from this saved blood can be used to treat disease that occurs later in that newborn's life with 100% matching safety. Usually thrown away with the after matter of birth, these pluripotent cells can be of inestimable value, especially for families with a history of stem cell—treatable disease.

Using stem cells to build or repair diseased or damaged organs is one pathway toward regeneration. Another, much further along in terms of clinical use, is what we call regenerative engineering. It is a true convergence of technologies that we can utilize for the purposes of regeneration of complex tissues.

This is a field I have been working in for more than 25 years. My laboratory, along with several others in the United States and abroad, has been at the forefront in developing therapies based on repairing and generating human body structures from patients' own cells. The work is still evolving, and we learn new things every day. At our University of Connecticut's Institute for Regenerative Engineering, our own grand challenge right now is regenerating a full and functioning human limb.

Why This? Why Now?

One of the most difficult of surgical endeavors is the repair of severely damaged or diseased limbs. Just think, nearly 200,000 people undergo upper or lower limb amputation every year. There are two million people in this country who live with limb loss in the United States. And then, there are the disparities—Black Americans are nearly four times as likely to undergo an amputation than their white counterparts.

When surgeons are unable to salvage a limb, and they have to amputate, the current medical solution is the use of a prosthetic. There is a lot of excitement these days about robotics and artificial appendages, and robotics do significantly increase functionality and capability. But they do this at an extremely high cost, and for all the advances, mechanical prosthetics will never be capable of reproducing the comfort, efficacy, and simple naturalness of the real thing.

The need for limb regeneration is even more heightened right now because of wars we have had in Iraq and Afghanistan. In wounded soldiers returning from these conflicts, we have seen an inordinate percentage of limb injuries. The reason for this is that while head wounds are often fatal, soldiers now wear sophisticated armor that protects the body core. If soldiers do not die from their wounds, the chances are that they have a limb injury. As a result, the number of these injuries has risen exponentially. But it isn't just happening on the world's battlefields.

A parallel phenomenon has taken place on our roads. Car accidents are a leading cause of domestic injury. In earlier times, hospitals did not see that many major musculoskeletal car accident injuries. If you had an injury like that, you were probably dead. However, with the advent of airbags, people survive, but often with severe limb trauma that can lead to the need for amputation.

These and other injuries and diseases leading to amputation make the need for full limb regeneration a critical priority. Musculoskeletal regenerative engineering holds out the promise that we can meet this challenge. The question is How? The answer is using all the tools we have to bear and everything we have learned to date to create new and cutting-edge solutions.

The potential for regenerative engineering has been around for more than half a century, ever since Katherine Sanford, who was a researcher at the National Cancer Institute for nearly 50 years, demonstrated that it was possible to sustain and grow cells outside the body. Researchers who followed in her footsteps developed simplified mediums that allowed scientists to grow cells efficiently, which made possible the creation and wide distribution of cultured cells, which in turn opened new horizons for biomedical science. The national best seller, *The Immortal Life of Henrietta Lacks*, by Rebecca Skloot, has introduced many general readers to the story of cell life outside the human body and to the vast benefits that have resulted, the first of which was the creation of the Salk polio vaccine in 1955.

When I started working on my graduate studies in chemical engineering at MIT, the great scientist Robert Langer was already working with cells and drugs implanted on materials that degraded naturally. He was taking polymer-based materials, whose chemical makeup resulted in their eventual dissolution, and placing medications on them with the object of using these materials as delivery systems for drugs. He believed that if the material was engineered properly, the medications implanted and inserted them into patients' bodies at the site of, say, a tumor, and the medication would be released in dosages and over time periods that could be tuned according to the rate of breakdown of the polymer, which in the end would itself be completely dissolved away. Langer's work in this area led to the development of Gliadel, the first FDA-approved delivery system of drugs to tumors, in this case certain brain cancers. It should be noted that scientists like Langer have many projects in the pipeline at any one time. After the FDA approved Gliadel, he went on to take the lead at a little pharma company you may have heard of—Moderna that delivered COVID-19 vaccines to millions of Americans.

A Game Changer for Me

As an entering graduate student, I was advised to go see Dr. Langer, who is a chemical engineer. He's doing brilliant work, I was told, and he's an exceptional human being on top of it. Every Saturday he volunteers with kids in the cancer ward at Boston Children's Hospital. After I had talked to Langer for a bit, I got excited about the possibilities and decided that I had to study with him.

I must admit that I did not initially understand everything he was telling me about his research, but I felt that this was a person I needed to work with and learn from. Fortunately, for me, he agreed and showed me the place at his lab bench where I would be sitting while we worked on projects, the primary one being the Gladiel drug delivery system. Gladiel later would become a groundbreaking product used in treating malignant brain tumors.

In 1987, I had entered MIT as part of a joint Harvard-MIT MD/PhD program. It was a perfect fit for me, because early along in my medical school rotations I had decided that I wanted to be an orthopaedic surgeon. Over time, I discovered that I was good with my hands. I had big hands, good for the hammers, drills, saws, and retractors that are the tools of the orthopaedic surgeon's trade.

Then, at some time during my third-year surgery rotation, a sports medicine doctor said, "I need someone to go with me to Foxboro Stadium to examine the football players." In 2002, Foxboro Stadium was demolished and was replaced by Gillette Stadium.

"You may also have to go with me next weekend and stand on the sidelines during the game." When he asked for volunteers, my hand shot up. Spending that time at Foxboro working with professional football players settled it for me. As a doctor, orthopaedic surgery was what I was going to do. While both orthopaedic surgeons and sports medicine physicians are trained in musculo-skeletal medicine, sports medicine physicians do not specialize in surgery. In fact, despite what most people think, 90% of sports injuries do not call for surgeries.

Getting this opportunity to learn about the treatment and prevention of sports injury opened a completely new world for me. And it was a great accompaniment to my decision to become an orthopaedic surgeon. This opportunity to explore both sides of sports medicine was the perfect match. Being able to provide comprehensive medical care for athletes, sports teams, or active individuals who are simply looking to maintain a healthy lifestyle was a tremendous learning experience.

Starting My Own Lab

Later, when I was in the final stages of my PhD work, MIT offered me an instructor's position and a start-up laboratory. When I asked Dr. Langer's advice about what research he thought might be most worthwhile, he said, "You're going to be an orthopaedic surgeon. You should study bone and cartilage. For chemical engineering, those are new areas. No one's done that yet." The challenge was set.

This was in the late 1980s. Orthopaedic surgeons at that point were working almost entirely with materials that are hard and durable: bone grafts, joint replacements, screws, other fasteners, and metal plates. But with my background in engineering in material science, I could see the ways we could bridge the gaps by bringing together chemistry and orthopaedics surgery. This was a new way of thinking. And there were naysayers in the field who couldn't see the potential, who told me that it didn't make sense. They were sure that was not the direction orthopaedic research was moving in at that time. As an example, according to them, the use of degradable polymers—the area of my PhD studies—would not be at all promising in terms of productivity, career advancement, or clinical applicability in the orthopaedic world.

But despite the well-meaning advice, I decided to follow my own instincts. I knew I wanted to study how bone cells grew on degradable surfaces and saw how it had the potential to improve outcomes. I was driven to understand, in detail, how living cells and synthetic materials interact. I had the feeling that this would be a new and important area, and that the applications for orthopaedics were going to come, even if they were not here now.

What I had in mind was that if I could culture bone cells on degradable material, maybe I could coax the cells to grow into bone tissue, and then, taking a page from Dr. Langer's book, I could find a way to implant them in the body. If I succeeded with that, the material would degrade, and the patient would have new bone—replacing the diseased or crushed or absent bone that was the problem. Each step of that would be an immense challenge. No one had done it before. I knew I was stepping off a cliff into the unknown. But it was exciting and had the potential to change the way we practice medicine, and the way we improve the quality of life for so many patients.

Piecing the Puzzle

That concept, the replacement of bone tissue, was my goal, but first I had to find out if I could actually grow bone cells. To do that I needed a grant to fund the project, so I applied to the National Science Foundation (NSF) for my very first research grant. I believed that I was on to something and was excited to submit the proposal. This was pioneering work that I was embarking on. I truly believed that we were on the cusp of something important. Yet, when my grant proposal was reviewed, the comments came back positive, but far from encouraging.

After all, it had only been a few years since researchers had learned how to grow cells on any synthetic surface. According to NSF grant reviewers, the idea of growing bone cells on degradable materials was overly ambitious at the least. And Even though they didn't believe it would work, they agreed to let me go ahead and try.

As I continued my research and continued to be funded over time, I began focusing on how to regenerate tissue in a three-dimensional rather than a two-dimensional way. I had already succeeded in developing the material growing bone cells on certain biodegradable materials. The cells proliferated and spread out across the polymer surfaces I had discovered. But bone is three dimensional, not two dimensional. To engineer bone, I needed a three-dimensional structure that the cells would grow on, not a flat surface. I had to create a scaffolding or matrix that would support bone cell growth, allow the bone cells to knit together into tissue, and then, eventually, dissolve away.

After a good deal of trial and error, my team and I discovered that putting the polymer material into an emulsifier caused it to break down. If we stopped that process at a certain point, what we got was a block of polymer with holes in it. If we stopped it at different points, we would get different sized holes, or pores—that cells could grow into.

Then one of my graduate students took the thought process a step further. If we let the emulsification process go on until the end, what we were left with was a lot of little polymer microspheres. He suggested that we could let it all break down into the microspheres. Then we could isolate the microspheres and bond them together to create any size pores we wanted. If it worked, we could then build a three-dimensional structure with exactly the openings that would be most conducive to cell growth. It worked and that was what we did.

Working with our manufactured matrices, we were able to determine what it takes to make cells go into a pore, showing why and under what conditions they do that.

If it sounds like a complex concept, it is. But one way to envision this is to think what you might do if you were walking down the street and came to a hole in the pavement. The chances are that you would walk around it. But if the hole was extremely wide, maybe half a block wide, you might be more likely to want to walk through it. As it turns out, assuming the depth is pretty manageable, a hole with a width that is about ten times your height is something you might look at to go through rather than around.

That is a concept that is true for cells, as well. The average cell is 10 microns in diameter. A 100–150 microns is the size of a hole that makes a cell want to go into it rather than around it. Once we knew that, we were able to engineer our polymer microspheres so that they presented bone cells with the most conducive openings, which meant that we were now able to create bone from patients' own cells (Fig. 1.1).

The Next Adventure

In this world of research, there is always the next challenge, or "what if," when it comes to discoveries that lead to solutions. Medical researchers, scientists, and engineers are at their core problem solvers. It is how we keep bringing developments that benefit patients moving forward to the fore. But it should be noted that there is success even when things don't work exactly as we plan. Of course, in science, as in life, we learn a lot about a process when it works the way we think it should. But in truth, we can learn as much about the processes and pivots when our research shows flaws that send us back to the drawing board, as when it works perfectly. Either way, we keep going. It is what we do.

Always Keep Your Eyes Open and Don't Be Afraid to Walk Through the Door

After I and my team made headway on the cell research, I started getting interested in the impact that our findings could have specifically on ligaments. By then, I was a new professor at Drexel University, and one day, I was walking past the lab of an acclaimed material science professor named Frank Ko. We had never met, but as I walked by his door was opened and he was standing just inside.

After we had introduced ourselves, he showed me a fiber of some sort. "What do you think about this?" he asked as he handed it to me. I took it and flexed it. It broke in my hands. "Not much," I said. "I don't think much of it."

His eyes lit up. "Okay. What do you think about this?" he said, then handing me a metal bar. "Well, it's a metal bar. What's the lesson in this?" I didn't get it.

He corrected me quickly. "No, it's not a metal bar. I made this bar with this same fiber I just gave you."

While the fiber itself was flexible, but weak, the bar was rigid and strong. I couldn't begin to break it. I found out later that Frank Ko originally made the crossbars for parasailing, which require a material very light and very strong.

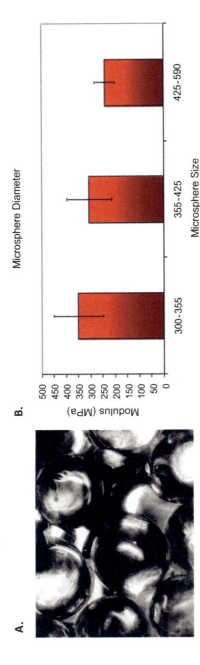

FIGURE 1.1 (A) Light microscopy image, microsphere fabrication. Characterized by a uniform microsphere shape and smooth surface. Microsphere size controlled by polymer concentration, stirring speed, and surfactant concentration. (B) Diameter optimization, microsphere diameters—300–355 μm, 355–425 μm, and 425–590 μm. *Presentation on Light Microsopy from Dr. Laurencin.*

Connecting the Dots

Even though I was at Drexel as a chemical engineering professor by then, I was also a practicing orthopaedic surgeon, specializing in sports medicine. In my practice I was seeing a lot of anterior cruciate ligament sprains or tears, known as an ACL.

Athletes who participate in high demand sports such as soccer, football, and basketball are more likely to injure their ACLs. If you have injured your ACL, you may require surgery to regain full function of your knee. The approach to the repair depends on several factors, such as the severity of your injury and your activity level. According to the Centers for Disease Control and Prevention (CDC), ACL injury affects as many as 250,000 individuals in the United States annually, resulting in healthcare costs that can exceed $2 billion a year. Globally, it is estimated that there are close to a million ACL injuries diagnosed each year.

In my practice, I thought that somewhere between fiber and this "metal" I had seen in Dr. Ko's lab is an ACL, say more somewhere between a fiber that's not strong but superflexible and this rigid, strong thing. So, I asked: How do you build strength into this fiber? It took doing a deep dive into textile 101 and asking how we take a single fiber and make it strong.

Essentially, the way you do that is by braiding. It turned out that there is actually a whole science of braiding, with which you can calculate and design the strength of a material based on the density of the braid, the size of the braid, and the angles between the individual braids. In Frank Ko's lab, he did that. He literally had a three-dimensional braiding machine that he used to design and make polymer and other kinds of fabric materials for various applications.

Once my team and I learned the science of the braiding, through our collaboration with Dr. Ko's team, we modeled a braid that had the precise flexibility and strength properties of an ACL. Then we took polymeric fibers—degradable fibers—and put them on a braiding machine, as if it were a regular textile. Through this collaboration, we were able to build an engineered ACL. Previously, surgeons would take the ACL out and replace it but they would eventually fail.

Learning from Others

We were not the first researchers to try to do this. A decade earlier, orthopaedic surgeons had used Dacron polyesters and Gortex to create prosthetic ACL grafts. Unfortunately, their artificial ACLs had failed miserably. After a year, patients were doing well with their repair. But then the materials used in the repair began to break down, and by 3 years out, they had fatigued completely and torn away, leaving the patients in considerable pain and distress. It was a common problem that required a solution.

I knew I wasn't interested in making an artificial ACL. What I wanted to do was to create an actual ACL from the patient's own cells, using matrix technology. We now knew how to make an ACL matrix—the braided polymers, and we knew what pore size was best for inducing cell growth.

Studying these kinds of material and cell interactions, we became better versed in the art of guiding cell behavior. We learned how to induce cells to reproduce and lay themselves down in the kind of orderly lines we needed them to do on the fibers of our braided matrix.

In a sense, here cells behaved as a human being might, say, if someone was trying to get you to walk on a plank stretched across the Grand Canyon. If that plank was 4 feet wide, your instinct would be to get down on all fours or on your belly and clutch onto that plank for dear life. The last thing you would want to do would be to move. But what if the plank was 25 feet wide? In that case, you might say to yourself, this is a little crazy, I'm over the Grand Canyon, but I can get up. I can walk. I can even run. If it looks like a highway and drive over it. If you have a mesh that is 1/10th your size, 25 ft wide I can.

Let's put it another way. If a braided matrix is engineered to the right specifications, cells can do the same thing. They like the environment; they're comfortable with it. They're happy to become mobile and proliferate. They link together and work up and down the line. The diameter and the tilt you've engineered induce them to do what you want them to do. In a patient, a torn ACL leaves its stumps anchored into bone on either side of the knee joint. Implanting a braided ACL matrix induces the patient's ACL cells to grow from the stumps onto the matrix and to proliferate and knit together with each other. When this process is complete, the matrix material degrades and, finally, washes away, leaving the patient with a new ACL created wholly out of his or her own ligament tissue.

Engineering a real ACL had been in the work of years. As of this writing, we have successfully completed animal trials. We know that the process works on rabbits and sheep which have ACLs that are similar to humans. Now we are currently in human trials. This research is significant because the need is so great. And as people stay active longer and look for quality of life and greater mobility, we can keep people moving. Each year orthopaedic surgeons reconstruct over 350,000 torn ACLs in the United States alone. To do this, they currently use either cadaver ligaments or tendons taken from the patient's own patellar or hamstring tendons.

The work we are doing in the lab today with regenerative engineering has the potential to revolutionize the art of successful ACL surgery. I believe it will, and that the human trials we are undertaking will be as successful as the animal trials have been (Fig. 1.2).

While we work on the ACL trials, our Institute has been able to engineer the other types of tissue that are found in the limbs: tissue for muscles, tendons, nerves, skin, and blood vessels. Work on these has been an outgrowth of our original work on bone and ligaments.

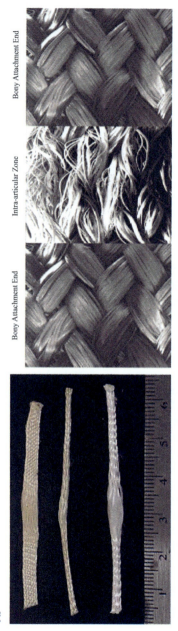

FIGURE 1.2A Engineered ligament. Degradable, three-dimensional (3-D) braided poly-L-lactic acid (PLLA) scaffold. Controlled pore size, Integrated pores, wear and rupture resistance, mechanical properties comparable with natural ACL and hierarchical design. *Presentation from Dr. Laurencin.*

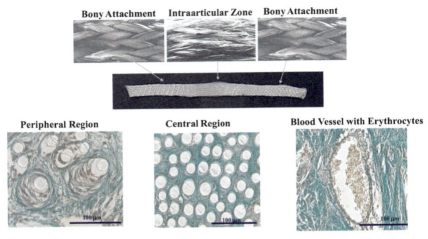

FIGURE 1.2B   Laurencin labs. Seeded PLA tissue-engineered ligament (12 weeks) after implantation. *Presentation from Dr. Laurencin.*

As we were making steady progress on creating the various types of limb tissue, new items began appearing on the advances in prosthetic technology for arms. Efforts were being made to develop artificial limbs that simulated the major types of upper limb movements and that were controlled by the patient's own musculature. Much of this robotic and prosthetic research was being driven by the desire to help returning combat veterans who had lost limbs.

These developments offer significant potential. The new mechanical arms were able to perform a variety of common tasks, lifting a cup, for example, and it was fascinating watching the bionic movements mimic a number of natural movements. But this kind of thing didn't seem like a satisfying solution to me.

For researchers like me, there are always new questions—many involving how we can achieve better outcomes for our patients. No matter how advanced the robotics have become, amputees were still going to be left with a prosthesis that was cumbersome and would never be capable of the finely nuanced control and tactile sensitivity they had enjoyed previous to their injury. The ideal long-term solution would be to give amputees the ability to reconstitute their own natural limbs. As fantastic and futuristic as this may have seemed five years ago, through synergy across research areas we are working to make this a reality.

Like Dr. Langer and the many professionals that I have had the privilege of working with, I never rest on my laurels. There is much at stake for those who need these solutions. Our laboratory team began thinking seriously about the fact that we already had in our repertoire the technology to generate the various tissues incorporated in limbs. But rather than looking at these piecemeal, in terms of therapies for specific orthopaedic problems, what if we saw them as elements of a whole that we might be able to build into something complete in and of itself? The tissue we already knew how to make are the individual elements of a limb. We asked ourselves why not attempt to actually assemble them into a limb?

Human upper and lower extremities—limbs—are exceptionally complex structures. Simultaneously regenerating and integrating the many different tissue types that go into them is an almost unimaginable challenge. But we have important technologies available to pursue this goal, and, looking back, these technologies themselves were unimaginable 20 years ago What's necessary in this endeavor is to bring to bear all the understanding we have in the various areas of regenerative medicine. These include chemical engineering/material science, cell science, and developmental biology.

We have made tremendous advances in understanding how to engineer the interaction of cells and materials so that they work together to create different types of tissues. The response of cells, especially stem cells, to advanced biomaterials is in the forefront of our efforts. Our team is currently working to engineer materials so that they influence and guide how stem cells differentiate into the desired types of tissue. To do this, we are using matrices made of nanofibers and new kinds of polymers in ways that stimulate particular kinds of responses. We are always looking for ways to do it better.

These developments, which are building on two decades of work with cells and degradable materials, constitute what you might call a top-down approach to tissue and organ regeneration—top-down in the sense that scientists are precipitating and steering the regenerative process. We are also bringing to bear a bottom-up approach, and discovering and attempting to harness the body's intrinsic regenerative abilities. This is the role of developmental biology, more specifically, regenerative biology (Fig. 1.3).

We are Not Newts

Certain vertebrates, newts, for example, are capable of spontaneously regenerating a number of body parts, including limbs. If a newt loses a leg, in a relatively short time a new leg will grow to replace the old one (Fig. 1.4).

Intact tissues will assemble themselves from differentiated, highly prolific cells in some ways similar to how embryos develop from a mass of pluripotent cells into differentiated cells that follow a programmed schema of integrated growth. We are, needless to say, not newts. But even as adults, we retain vestiges of regenerative capability. Understanding what these are, how they work, and how they can be utilized is part of the arsenal we need to marshal as we pursue our grand challenge (Fig. 1.5).

The regeneration of a limb is what I think of as New World Engineering. We are, in this endeavor, exploring a new world, as if we were going to Mars. No one has done it before, but we have created many of the tools necessary to do it, and if we are intelligent enough, creative enough, and persistent enough, there's a good chance that eventually we will indeed get there.

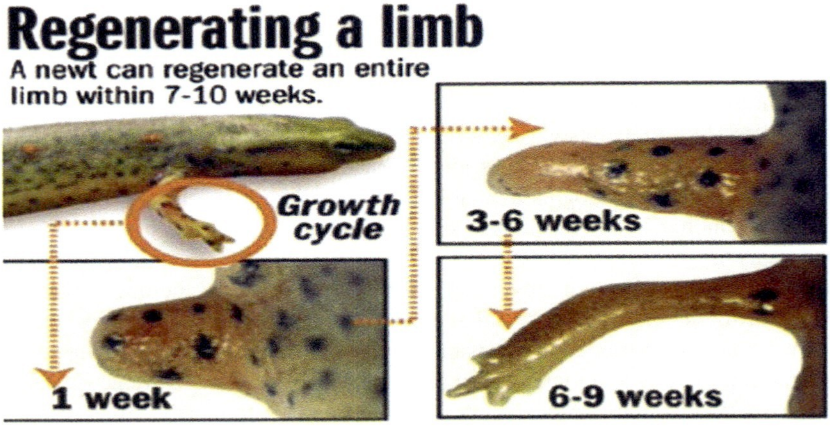

Regenerating a limb

A newt can regenerate an entire limb within 7-10 weeks.

Growth cycle

3-6 weeks

1 week

6-9 weeks

FIGURE 1.3 Bottom-up approach—tissues assembled from the cellular scale and up to produce fully intact tissue structures. Translational challenges—many, but must be part of the arsenal.

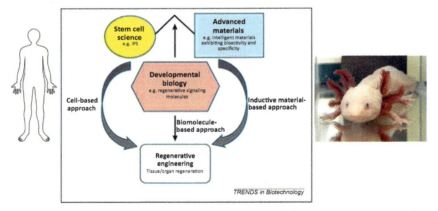

FIGURE 1.4 The grand challenge in regenerative engineering is to identify the regeneration-enabling signals from axolotl to the improvement of human repair mechanisms. GRID is a novel tool for complex tissue regeneration in mammals. *From Lo, K.W.-H., Jiang, T., Gagnon, K.A., Nelson, C., Laurencin, C.T., 2014. Trends in Biotechnology 32(2): 74-81.*

Top scientists and researchers in the field are often asked to present on their work and innovations. Over the years, I have done countless presentations. When I first articulated this idea about regeneration of limbs in 2010 at a Summit on Grand Challenges, very few people in the scientific world thought it was a possibility. Now years later, as research evolves at an increasingly rapid pace, we can see medical and scientific opinion shifting. I believe that

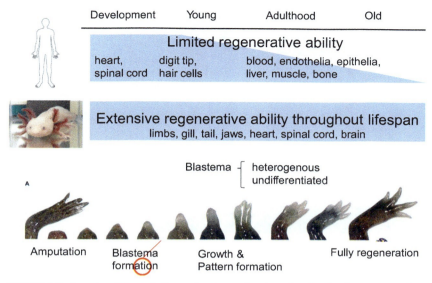

FIGURE 1.5   Learning from axolotls to enhance complex tissue regeneration in mammals. *From McCusker, C., Bryant, S.V., Gardiner, D.M., 2015. Regeneration 2(2):54-71.*

what is often thought of as impossible dreams can begin to look increasingly like coming reality.

I'd like to share a presentation I made about our work to date and a glimpse about our plans for the future.

"Thank you. It is really an honor and pleasure to be here today to receive this award and to give my lecture. I am honored that the award recognizes our work on complex tissue regeneration, an area where we are accomplishing groundbreaking basic and applied science for the benefit of people. I am Dr. Cato Laurencin and I am very honored to be able to provide a lecture today on regenerative engineering, A Convergence Approach for Addressing Grand Challenges. At the University of Connecticut, I am the University Professor and the Albert and Wilda Van Dusen distinguished endowed professor of Orthopaedic Surgery. I am a professor of chemical and biomolecular engineering, professor of material science and engineering, and professor of biomedical engineering at UConn. I am the chief executive officer of the Connecticut Convergence Institute for Translation and Regenerative Engineering with laboratories on both the medical campus and the engineering campus. At the Connecticut Convergence Institute our main focus is on regenerative engineering, which as I mentioned is defined as the convergence of advanced materials sciences, stem cell science, physics, developmental biology, and clinical translation, for the regeneration of complex tissues and organ systems (Fig. 1.6)."

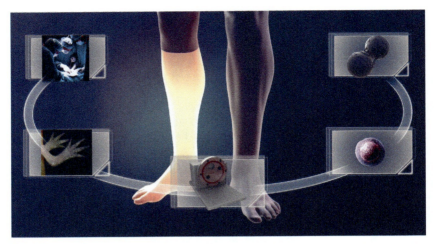

FIGURE 1.6 The convergence of advanced materials sciences, stem cell science, physics, developmental biology, and clinical translation, for the regeneration of complex tissues and organ systems. Embedded in this new field includes the following five areas: (1) advanced materials sciences, (2) stem cell sciences, (3) physics, (4) developmental biology, and (5) clinical translation.

Our Institute aims to regenerate human limbs, not robotic limbs but rather real, organic, flesh-and-blood ones that grow on the person receiving treatment. This type of breakthrough will have a tremendous impact on global public health and in the lives of those with amputations due to bone cancer, diabetes, dangerous infections, trauma accidents, or children born with missing or impaired limbs.

These are some of my relevant disclosures. I'll talk about products involving companies that I own, lead, direct, receive royalties from or conduct clinical trials with, including Soft Tissue Regeneration, Globus Medical, Bio Bind, Healing Orthopaedic Technologies, MiMedics, HOT Bone, and others along the way.

The area of tissue engineering has been defined in a number of ways. I've defined it as the application of biological, chemical, and engineering principles toward the repair restoration or regeneration of living tissues using biomaterials, cells, and factors alone or in combination.

Earlier this year, I was speaking to a group of trainees during a virtual Visiting Professor Day, who were graduate students and postdoctoral fellows. One of the trainees said, "I want to ask you a question, Professor, and please don't take any offense." Obviously, whenever on a virtual call and someone says please don't take any offense to start with, I'm always concerned. But she said respectfully, "This area of tissue engineering, we were hoping to have lots of grand challenges that were met, and we've had some progress in the area, but we really haven't met a lot of grand challenges."

I agree with this person that the area of tissue engineering itself, in terms of being able to meet the types of grand challenges that we've wanted to have and create the science and technologies we've wanted to see, has not really accomplished things in the way that we'd like. In fact, the editors of Science Translational Medicine actually asked me a few years ago about my vision for the future of engineering tissues. What I said was that our traditional way of thinking about tissue engineering is okay, but if we really want to solve grand challenges and really in fact move forward, we need to rethink how we approach engineering tissues. In that piece in Science Translational Medicine, I really spoke to the fact that we need to create a new field that I call regenerative engineering. Basically, I said that the future of tissue regeneration lies in this area of regenerative engineering.

Regenerative engineering is a convergence discipline. By convergence, we mean the coming together of insights and approaches from originally distinct fields. Our goal is to bring together areas that are distinct and may not seem to fit in and bring them together to be able to solve problems such as complex tissue regeneration.

So, these areas that we work in are in advanced material science including nanotechnology, the use of stem cells and stem cell science, physics, and physical forces, including bioreactor work, developmental biology, and morphogenesis, how a newt or salamander regenerates a limb. But it's also very important to integrate clinical translation. This includes how regeneration takes place in the clinician's eyes and how we can utilize knowledge and experience from immunology and other patient factors to allow regeneration to take place. Much of our work has focused on the regeneration of musculoskeletal tissues. I'm a material scientist and a chemical engineer, but I'm also an orthopaedic surgeon. I'm a shoulder and knee surgery surgeon, so a lot of my work is focused on shoulder and knee research.

Our beginning work was on engineering a bone with our ultimate goal to create a biodegradable porous polymer matrix that will allow for bone regeneration to take place.

We start with synthesizing and fabricating degradable polymeric microspheres. We could characterize these by uniform microsphere size and shape. We could do some nice material science and engineering in terms of the creation of these polymeric microspheres by controlling polymer concentration, stirring speed, and surfactant concentration in designing emotion systems for microsphere creation (Fig. 1.7).

As we heat these polymeric microspheres above the glass transition temperature of the polymer, we can create centered microsphere matrices. For the microsphere matrices, we can vary the diameter of the spheres. By doing so, we can modulate the mechanical properties of these microsphere matrices when they're centered based upon the size of the microspheres.

These centered microsphere matrices come in a variety of shapes and sizes. They can be used in a variety of different settings. In one experiment, we

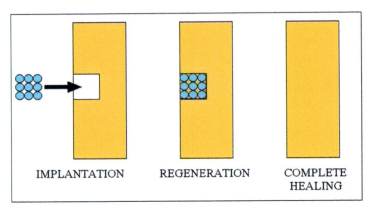

FIGURE 1.7 Regenerative engineering of bone. The ultimate goal is to create a biodegradable, porous matrix that allows for bone regeneration to take place.

utilized an in vivo ulnar defect model of the rabbit. We like this model for a number of reasons. Number one, we can create a critical size defect, meaning that without the use of a morphogenetic material, it will not heal. The second is the fact that we have the radius on the other side.

It's an internal structure. This obviates the use of a plate fixation for the area. If you squint, you can see the microspheres that are in the matrix. We could implant it in the deep defect area of the ulna. This is what we see after 8 weeks. This is with our microsphere matrix along with a bone morphogenetic protein, BNP7 in this case, and also marrow that's actually absorbed onto the matrix. We see a robust amount of bone formation taking place around the areas of the microspheres (Fig. 1.8).

We've utilized this concept of the engineered microsphere matrix (Fig. 1.9).

It's inspired a number of products, including the microfused product that's developed by Globus Medical, for which I have received royalties (Fig. 1.10).

It's great to experience times in which we've sketched out a problem and a possible solution, then worked on that problem from the basic research, applied research, and clinical translation standpoints to create real technologies that actually then go into humans and actually help people.

Another area that I've been involved is examining the nanoscale mechanisms and the nanoscale for regeneration. Now, there's some natural appeal in terms of the use of the nanoscale materials. The increased surface area to volume provides more sites for cellular adhesion. In general, the nanoscale environment creates a more biomimetic environment. We have a slide on an osteoblast on a microscale film, and an osteoblast on the nanoscale film. We can see the differences that take place in terms of these surface areas (Fig. 1.11).

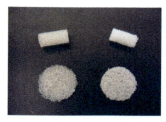 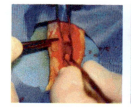 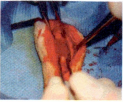

FIGURE 1.8   Left image: Sintered scaffolds. Right image: In vivo—rabbit ulnar defect model.

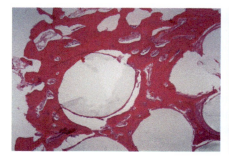 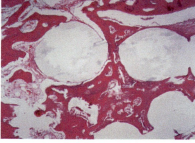

FIGURE 1.9   Histological bone sections of matrix + BMP + marrow-derived cells at 8 weeks. Histological results show bone growth within the matrix.

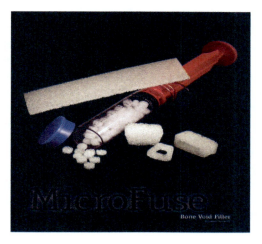

FIGURE 1.10   Engineered bone matrix—MicroFuse.

Osteoblasts on microscale film   **Osteoblasts on nanoscale film**

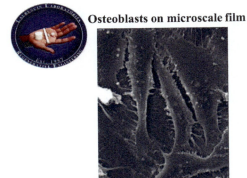 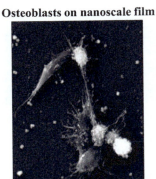

FIGURE 1.11   Nanoscale mechanisms. Increased surface area to volume ratio provides more sites for adhesion protein. Nanoscale creates a more biomimetic environment and allows for focal adhesion areas which aid the osteoblast in maintaining phenotype.

We were very fortunate to write the first paper in the refereed literature showing the suitability of using nanofiber matrices, polymeric nanofiber matrices, for the engineering of tissues. It has had approximately 2800 citations, so far (Fig. 1.12).

I started working in the area of using electrospun and nanofiber materials for engineering different tissues along with my colleague, Professor Frank Ko. The paper I just mentioned was selected for cover story in the 100th volume of the *Journal of Biomedical Materials Research* and recognized in the top 25 papers in the literature during the past 50 years. My students told me that this means because it made the cover, that it was the number one paper in the past 50 years. I'm not going to argue with them on that, but it was really a landmark paper using polymer nanofibers for different technology for regeneration.

There are a number of ways in which we can use nanofiber materials for regenerative purposes. One is in the area of the skin. Approximately 400,000 burn injuries take place each year, and nearly 4000 patients still die in terms of burn injuries each year in America. Internationally, over 180,000 people die each year of burns. Autografts are of limited supply and have potential donor site morbidity. Allografts have a risk of immunological rejection and also a risk of disease transmission.

We performed a number of studies involving nanofiber technology for skin. In one of our first studies, we utilized the same polymeric material, polylactic acid, and glycolic acid material and examined the growth of human skin fibroblasts on these different matrices, with the only difference in the matrices being the diameter of the materials. What we have seen is that in the nano-regime, we can modulate the growth and also modulate the differentiation of cells just using sizes in the nano regime (Fig. 1.13).

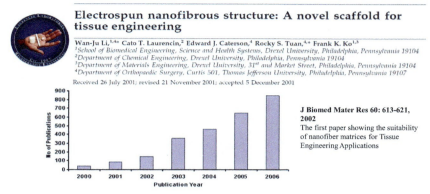

Electrospun nanofibrous structure: A novel scaffold for tissue engineering

Wan-Ju Li,[1,4a] Cato T. Laurencin,[2] Edward J. Caterson,[4] Rocky S. Tuan,[4,*] Frank K. Ko[1,3]
[1]School of Biomedical Engineering, Science and Health Systems, Drexel University, Philadelphia, Pennsylvania 19104
[2]Department of Chemical Engineering, Drexel University, Philadelphia, Pennsylvania 19104
[3]Department of Materials Engineering, Drexel University, 31st and Market Street, Philadelphia, Pennsylvania 19104
[4]Department of Orthopaedic Surgery, Curtis 501, Thomas Jefferson University, Philadelphia, Pennsylvania 19107

Received 26 July 2001; revised 21 November 2001; accepted 5 December 2001

J Biomed Mater Res 60: 613-621, 2002
The first paper showing the suitability of nanofiber matrices for Tissue Engineering Applications

FIGURE 1.12   Nanofiber matrices. Growing number of publications in nanofiber and related applications.

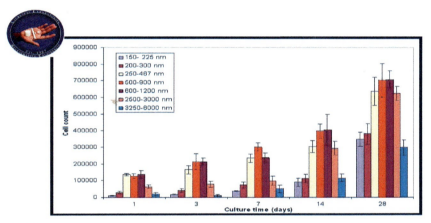

FIGURE 1.13   Human skin fibroblast growth modulated by nanofiber characteristics. Cell growth with nanofiber matrix size over 28 days.

Next, we explored the creation of matrices using nanofibers. We created nanomatrices and then compared with our microsphere matrices. We compared ectopic bone formation in mice using a nanomatrix versus a micromatrix. What we found was if we examine the nanomatrix versus the micromatrix, the nanomatrix actually made more bone (Fig. 1.14).

This was owing to our ability to be able to utilize the nanoregime, in terms of increasing the phenotypic expression of cells we believe.

We went on to create more of these nanomatrices specifically for bone regeneration. Our team found that the nanomatrices were not physically or mechanically competent enough to be able to be placed in a lot of different

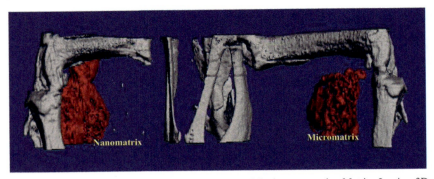

FIGURE 1.14 Ectopic bone formation in mice, nanoMatrix versus microMatrix. In vivo 3D micro-CT scans showing ectopic bone formation using nano- and microfiber matrices.

weight-bearing locations. We then decided to come up with another plan that incorporated nanofibers into our microsphere matrix and try to get the best of both worlds. We utilized our microsphere matrix and combined it with our nanofiber to a gel nanomethod to create microspheres and micro–nanomatrices. The microsphere component was utilized for its mechanical strength, while the nanocomponent was utilized for its ability to promote phenotypic expression.

Here, we see the sphere with our nanofibers that are present between the sphere areas. We've examined the performance of these micro–nanomatrices using polylactic acid and polyglycolic acid and another polymer that we've worked with that we'll talk about called polyphosphazenes. If we examine alkaline phosphatase expression, osteopontin expression, osteocalcin expression, and also scaffold calcification, we find that they're all enhanced when cells are attached to these nanofiber matrices in combination with a microsphere matrix. So, thinking about this from a regenerative engineering lens, we find the use of nanomaterials to be important in enhancing the phenotypic expression of cells seeded on the matrices.

Our work has also focused on hydroxyapatite. It's the main mineral component of bone. It's osteoconductive and binds directly to the bone. We were interested in creating polymer-reinforced composites that allowed us again to have the best of both worlds. The hydroxyapatite is brittle and has low tensile strength and low resistance to impact loading. Creating matrices that combine hydroxyapatite with polymeric materials would allow us to be able to have materials that have higher mechanical strength and impact loading capability.

We combined these polymeric materials with our ceramics to create polymer–ceramic composites for regeneration (Fig. 1.15).

Using a method that we've now patented in terms of creating these composite microspheres, we were able to create amorphous or low crystalline and calcium phosphate microspheres using polylactic acid and polyglycolic acid in

POLYMER (PLGA)	**CERAMIC (CaP)**
Strength, formability, ease of use, biodegradable	Bioactive, osteoconductive, osteointegrative
Limited osteoconductivity, osteointegration and bioactivity	Brittle in failure, poor formability, slow degradation

POLYMER/CERAMIC COMPOSITE
Biodegradable, formable, osteoconductive, osteointegrative material

FIGURE 1.15 Composite structures. Combined polymeric materials with our ceramics to create polymer—ceramic composites for regeneration.

much the same way as we created our polymeric microsphere emulsion systems (Fig. 1.16).

If we examine the mechanical properties of these systems, we find that we can modulate the mechanical properties by changing hydroxyapatite concentration, stirring speed, and stirring time and create materials that have really high strength in terms of compressive modulus and vary in their mechanical properties (Fig. 1.17).

At the same time, thinking about our regenerative engineering work, we began to explore the use of stem cell technologies for regeneration. We have adult, embryonic, and induced pluripotent stem cells. Our work has really involved adult stem cells. We believe that these are stem cells for all. We now have procedures to isolate our adult stem cells. For instance, we can isolate

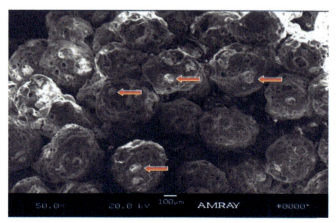

FIGURE 1.16 Composite microspheres. Amorphous or low crystalline and calcium phosphate microspheres created using polylactic acid and polyglycolic acid.

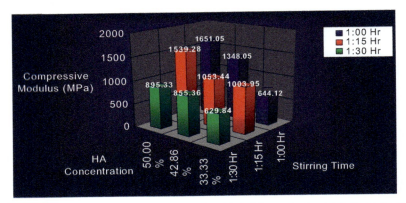

FIGURE 1.17   Microsphere mechanical properties. We find that we can modulate the mechanical properties by changing hydroxyapatite concentration, stirring speed and stirring time, and create materials that have really high strength in terms of compressive modulus and vary in their mechanical properties.

them in the operating room from the human infrapatellar fat pads from patients undergoing knee surgery. We can rapidly isolate and filter the materials to create populations of stem cells that we could now use and implant after isolation in the operating room. These cells can differentiate down a number of different lines, including bone as we've demonstrated in multiple papers.

One of the areas that we've explored, and I think that we've been one of the pioneers in, is in the area of inductive materials. The concept of inductive materials is that while the dogma is that in order to be able to have a cell differentiate, it has to be in the presence of an applied morphogenetic protein that's actually placed in the area. We believe with others that we can create materials that are actually inherently inductive that cause the differentiation of cells.

So, we start with our polymer and our ceramic to create these polymer—ceramic composite materials. Again, they are biodegradable, formable, osteoconductive, and osteointegrative. Of course, we can really modulate their mechanical properties. But, if we create these with low crystalline hydroxyapatite materials, we can then more precisely modulate the calcium and phosphate release from these materials. The modulation of the calcium and phosphate release allows us to be able to control cellular activity in terms of differentiation.

If we take adipose-derived stem cells, we can place them on our polymer—ceramic matrices that contain low crystalline hydroxyapatite with precise release of calcium and phosphate. This is a study done over 21 days. If we measure osteocalcin and BNP2 production, we find that osteocalcin and BNP2 production by these adipose-derived stem cells takes place, which is consistent with their cellular differentiation toward bone (Fig. 1.18).

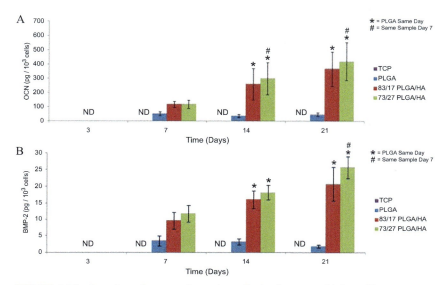

FIGURE 1.18 Secretion of osteogenic markers. Study done over 21 days. If we measure osteocalcin and BNP2 production, we find that osteocalcin and BNP2 production by these adipose-derived stem cells takes place, which is consistent with their cellular differentiation toward bone.

Again, if we examine in vitro mineralization of these materials using unseeded matrices versus seeded matrices with our low and high amounts of low crystalline hydroxyapatite, we can see increased scaffold calcification and mineralization taking place (Fig. 1.19).

Then finally, we can take this in vivo with our critical size defect model that we've talked about before and place our matrices. This is our microsphere matrix with the low crystalline polymer ceramic matrix along with adipose-derived stem cells. This is what we see after eight weeks. What we find in terms of the composite healing area, we see areas of new bone formation with new rimming bone in that area (Fig. 1.20A).

This is consistent with the differentiation of these adipose-derived cells of the bone without the use of exogenous morphogenetic factors.

The mechanism by which this is happening has been described by a number of individuals, including us, but mainly by Luyton where calcium phosphate—based biomaterials, if there are low crystalline, could release calcium and phosphate. Then there are a number of effects that can take place. There is a mitogenic effect that takes place with these cells. There's also regulation of extracellular matrix. But what is really fascinating is that there is a release of BNP2 that creates an autocrine—paracrine induction loop (Fig. 1.20B).

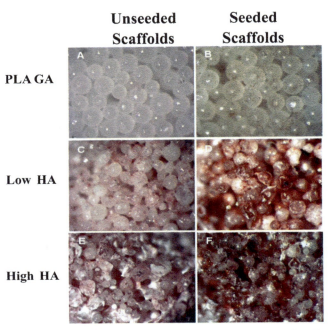

FIGURE 1.19 In vitro mineralization using unseeded matrices versus seeded matrices with low and high amounts of low crystalline hydroxyapatite, we can see increased scaffold calcification and mineralization taking place.

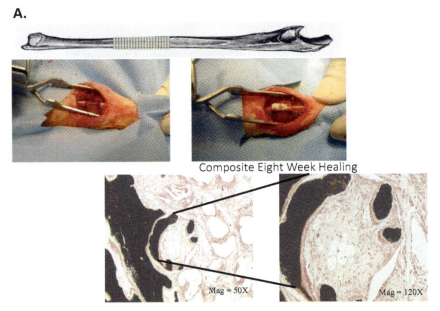

FIGURE 1.20A In vivo evaluation. Evidence of remodeling is seen after 8 weeks of healing in the callus of the composite scaffold. Multinucleated osteoclasts are seen along the border between fibrous tissue and mineralized tissue.

B.

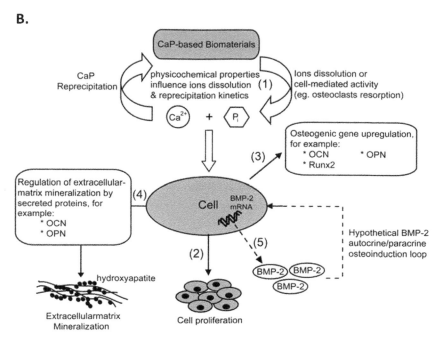

FIGURE 1.20B Osteoinductive calcium/phosphate ions (Luyten). Calcium phosphate−based biomaterials, if low crystalline, could release calcium and phosphate. There is a mitogenic effect that takes place with these cells. There's also regulation of extracellular matrix and a release of BNP2 that creates an autocrine−paracrine induction loop.

This is what we've demonstrated in the previous slides that could take place through our in vitro mechanistic studies. That's the main mechanism by which we seed bone.

We can perform direct comparative analysis of our micromatrix with our micro−nanomatrix. We utilize a mouse parietal bone defect model (Fig. 1.21).

We have our microsphere matrix on one side and our microsphere nanomatrix on the other side. This is what we can see over time. If we quantify using Alizarin complexone of our microsphere versus our micro−nanomatrix. For our microsphere matrix, we do see evidence of Alizarin complexone that's present. With our micro−nanomatrix, we really have an exuberant amount of Alizarin complexone that we can visually see expressed in the area (Fig. 1.22).

What happens when we combine this with low crystalline hydroxyapatite materials? We created a critical size cranial defect in the mouse. We have bilateral defects in the area. We actually in this case heated cells that have an origin with bone marrow, and we used a transgenic mouse host and donor model, Dr. David Rowe, where Topaz reports host collagen and Siam reports donor collagen production.

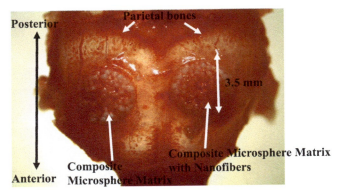

FIGURE 1.21 Bone regeneration using bone matrix. Direct comparative analysis of our micromatrix with our micro–nanomatrix. We utilize a mouse parietal bone defect model.

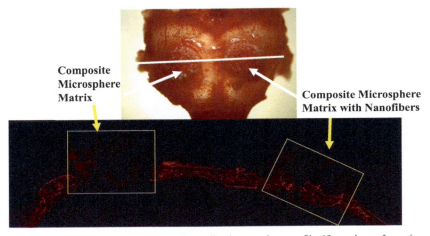

FIGURE 1.22 Bone quantification using Alizarin complexone. Significant bone formation: Alizarin complexone stain shows the two defects bound by host bone.

This picture is worth a thousand words. This is with everything combined, our micro–nanoceramic matrix. Our microsphere matrix provides us our mechanical strength. Our nanocomponent helps with our phenotypic expression. Our ceramic portion works in terms of differentiation due to low crystalline ceramic material. Here are microspheres that are present in the area. We have areas of new bone formation that's present (Fig. 1.23).

Then we have these donor cells that are in blue. They are coming from the matrix itself. We can see that they are laying down bone in these areas. We can also see areas of host bone coming in from the sides. In our published work, we have quantifiable information in these areas and have found significantly higher amounts of bone in our micro–nanoceramic systems.

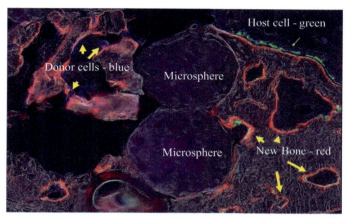

FIGURE 1.23   Micro–nanoceramic stem cell. Microspheres that are present in the area and new bone formation are present.

We are very positive about this microsphere micro–nanoceramic matrix combining the capabilities of mechanical properties, mechanical strength, and phenotypic expression, along with the ability to be able to differentiate cells. We are working actively to bring this next-generation technology to patients.

Our next area that we've worked in extensively is in the area of engineered ligament regeneration. For our work on engineered ligaments, we've concentrated on the anterior cruciate ligament of the knee. It's the major intraarticular ligament of the knee. It controls motion and acts as a stabilizer. ACL injuries can lead to excessive joint mobility and instability. So again, working with Dr. Frank Ko when he was with me at Drexel, we decided to use a new approach and to create three-dimensional braided systems for ACL regeneration.

I was very impressed one day when I walked into Dr. Ko's office and saw him working with some braided fabric and noted the ability to be able to obtain a wide range of mechanical properties with the braided fabric that I saw. With that in mind, we decided to work together to create a braided matrix that would be biomimetic for the ACL.

Now I'm going to summarize a number of years of work and a number of grad students and Fellows who have worked very, very hard. I also want to provide a shout-out to Dr. James Cooper who is a co-inventor on the patent of this ACL matrix. As it turns out, to create and engineer a ligament, you actually have to create two sets of tissues. Because ligaments connect bone to bone, then there is a soft tissue area in between. We had to create a bony attachment zone and an intraarticular zone, and then connect it to another bony attachment zone. We utilized three-dimensional braided polylactic acid with controlled pore size for cellular ingrowth and transport and controlled mechanical properties designed to mimic the natural ACL. We used the hierarchical design of the ACL to be able to mimic and create these matrices.

These efforts and wins don't happen overnight. Again, we're summarizing a number of years of work. For instance, one question that came up was what size should the diameter of the polymeric fibers be to allow for ACL cells to travel across the joint. As it turns out, the size is actually the size of the cell, about 10 microns. We studied a number of properties of cell transport on surfaces and published the paper on the dynamics of cell fiber interactions in the setting of regeneration. What we found was that if the cells were seeded onto fibers that had diameters on the order of a magnitude of its cell, they naturally traveled up and down those fibers. Cells seeded onto fibers in order of magnitude less than the cells take on a reticular pattern where they utilize the fibers as a trellis to hold onto. Cells seeded on areas in order of magnitude higher than the diameter of the cells actually exhibited Brownian motion on those surfaces.

The ability to be able to really control the dynamics of these cells is very important in terms of engineered regeneration. We created our three-dimensional matrix with a bony zone, intraarticular zone, and a bony zone. We then created a model in rabbits for regeneration of the ACL (Fig. 1.2).

This is what the ACL looks like after 3 months; we get a nice glistening ACL. During the 3-month period, the rabbits are running around and being happy and just being rabbits (Fig. 1.24).

This is what the histology of the matrix looks like after 12 weeks. We have the peripheral region. We have a central region. And in our peripheral region, we saw blood vessels with erythrocytes (Figs. 1.2 and 1.24).

Our ACL technology won the Nicholas Andry Award, which is the highest award of the Association of Bone and Joint Surgeons. Scientific American

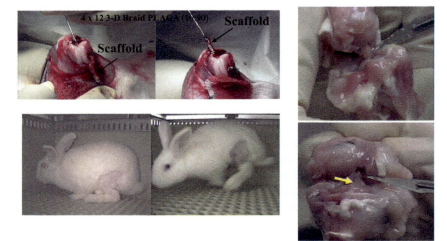

FIGURE 1.24 This is what the ACL looks like after 3 months, we get a nice glistening ACL. During the 3-month period, the rabbits are running around.

LC at 12 wks

6 Months ACL in
Sheep (1)

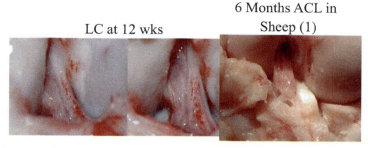

FIGURE 1.25   The L-C ligament, the Laurencin—Cooper ligament, at 12 weeks in a sheep model. We get a glistening ligament in sheep. Right image: the ligament at 6 months in sheep. After 2 years, we get regular dense collagen in tissue. We can now get complete regeneration of the ACL.

named it one of the 50 Greatest Scientific Achievements of the Year. But for me, it's still very, very memorable that I received a text from my Chemistry teacher in high school, Mr. William Brooks, as I landed from a flight from London. My Chemistry teacher never really thought I was going to be a scientist. I think he was always skeptical about my abilities. He actually texted me and said, "You're my greatest student ever, and I told everyone all of your achievements are because of me."

Later that day, he sent me an email that said that he was at his local Walgreens store and was browsing the magazines and picked up the National Geographic 100 Scientific Discoveries That Changed the World and found that our team listed under number 30. National Geographic magazine highlighted our work and the team that we had on creating an engineered ligament that provides a potential for allowing patients to recover more fully and allowing for complete regeneration of the ACL. To put this in perspective, space travel was ranked in the magazine as number 85. The cell phone was ranked number 15. Our placement under number 30 seems very appropriate.

From there, we scaled up the work in terms of larger animals and took it to a sheep model. This is the L-C ligament, the Laurencin-Cooper ligament, at 12 weeks. We get a glistening ligament in sheep. This is the ligament at 6 months in sheep. This is actually after 2 years that we get regular dense collagen in tissue. We know can get complete regeneration of the ACL (Fig. 1.25).

The Outcomes

So, using these principles of regenerative engineering, our engineered ligament has been implanted in people for over 6 years as of July 2020. The work has been very exciting and rewarding. Probably the most exciting and the most rewarding aspect of the work has been the work on ligament, but also the work

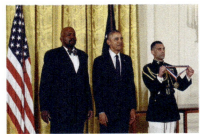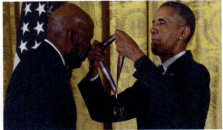

FIGURE 1.26   The L-C ligament, the Laurencin–Cooper ligament has been implanted in people for over 6 years as of July 2020. The work has been very exciting and rewarding. For this work I received the National Medal of Technology Innovation from President Barack Obama. It's the highest honor for technological achievement in the United States.

on bone. Equally exciting to the work was the fact that I received the National Medal of Technology Innovation from President Barack Obama. It's the highest honor for technological achievement in the United States. Pictures of Obama (Fig. 1.26).

I have. I was very proud to receive the National Medal of Technology. I was also very, very proud to receive it from President Obama, who's done so much in terms of working in science. Not to digress, but the other great thing about getting the award was the fact that it's actually a two-part award. In the afternoon, you have the award ceremony, but in the morning, you get to bring your family and meet and spend time with the President. This is probably the greatest part of the ceremony, the morning portion and spending time with the family and the President.

We Never Rest on What We've Accomplished

Well, the question is what's next after that? I remember driving back from Washington, and one of my children said, "Dad, what's next? You just won the National Medal of Technology and Innovation. Are you done?" And I said, no, we've got lots of more work to do and lots more areas to cover.

A lot of our work is now involved in addressing the rotator cuff tendon of the shoulder. Millions of people are living with rotator cuff tendon injuries. There are over 300,000 rotator cuff surgeries performed each year in the United States. If one looks at methods to regenerate and to reinforce the rotator cuff, there are a number of different materials, such as AlloPatch, CuffPatch, and Restore, but none of these have the mechanical properties of the infraspinatus tendon.

So, we went back to the lab and refined using polymeric nanofiber technology. We published the first paper on their use in tissue regeneration. We worked on the development of a nanofiber matrix that could be utilized and implanted for reinforcement and regeneration of the rotator cuff.

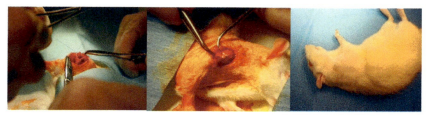

FIGURE 1.27 Surgical procedure of a rat model for the rotator cuff. Human shoulders are actually much like a rat shoulder, in terms of the mechanics and dynamics of the bony and soft tissue structures around it. We created an acute rotator cuff tear in the rat and then reinforced it with our matrix.

Our team chose a rat model for the rotator cuff because human shoulders are actually much like a rat shoulder, in terms of the mechanics and dynamics of the bony and soft tissue structures around it. We created an acute rotator cuff tear in the rat and then reinforced it with our matrix (Fig. 1.27).

What we found is that with primary repair, at four weeks, we had seven megapascals of strength that went down to less than four megapascals of strength after eight weeks. With our augmented matrix repair, it was at four megapascals at four weeks and then 48.6 megapascals of strength at eight weeks (Fig. 1.28).

This study published in the *Journal of Bone and Joint Surgery* demonstrated the great potential of these systems for rotator cuff regeneration. With this work, we were able to demonstrate that we can create nanofiber matrices that can really augment the repair and regeneration of rotator cuff.

Now, through a lens of regenerative engineering, we've taken on a different way of thinking about it. So instead of using the matrix as a physical soft tissue reinforcement, our new work has involved the use of stem cells to influence the regeneration of the native tendon itself.

	4 Weeks (MPa)	8 Weeks (MPa)
Primary Repair	7.2 ±3.8	3.79 ±2.1
Augmented Repair	4.0 ±0.5	48.6 ± 9.5

FIGURE 1.28 Mechanical properties of the rotator cuff augmentation device in vivo from the rat model. Nanofiber-augmented rotator cuff showed better mechanical performance compared with primary repair with time.

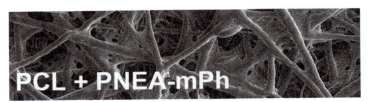

FIGURE 1.29 Combining two biodegradable polymers combines the beneficial characteristics of PCL and PNEA-mPh for the purpose of rotator cuff repair augmentation and MCS cell delivery.

We started with two polymeric materials, polycaprolactone and polyphosphazene materials, and brought them together (Fig. 1.29).

They have different strengths and weaknesses. As a blend, they end up having the ability to be able to combine beneficial characteristics for the purpose of rotator cuff repair and augmentation.

For instance, these are cells grown in three hours in cells culture with buffered saline (Fig. 1.30).

What we can see using the polycaprolactone material is that the cells are attaching. With our polyphosphazene materials as part of the blend, we find increased cell spreading and an increased number of cell processes. The use of a blend material in this area can be very beneficial.

We utilized our model in the rat for rotator cuff repair where we create and tear the rotator cuff, then we repair it. We also have a group where we create a tear and repair it with our matrix, and a group where we create a tear and repair it with our matrix along with bone marrow—derived stem cells (Fig. 1.31).

The first question is what's occurring at the tendon insertion? Because in general, when there are tears of the rotator cuff, clinically they take place at the tendon insertion. What we found was that cell seeding allowed us to have a morphology very similar to intact native tendon. On the top corner, we have native tendon. We have our repair group next to it. Next to it is the repair plus

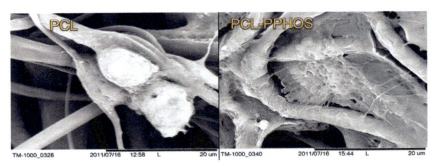

FIGURE 1.30 PNEA-MPH increases initial cell adhesion. Cells grown for 3 hours with buffered saline and polycaprolactone material the cells are attaching. With polyphosphazene materials as part of the blend, there are increased cell spreading and an increased number of cell processes.

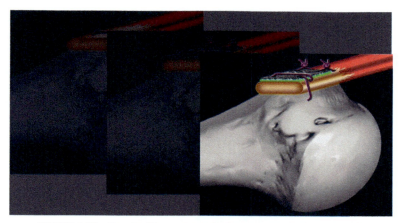

FIGURE 1.31 Rat shoulders were repaired or augmented w/ or w/o cells.

scaffold group. And our repair plus scaffold plus cells group is next to that. The repair plus scaffold plus cells group result is much more consistent with native tendon (Figs. 1.32 and 1.33).

The next question is what's happening also in the substance of the tendon. What we found was that cell seeding allowed for the tendon body remodeling to take place. This is the intact tendon with repair. Our repair plus scaffold shows improvement over repair. But our sole scaffold matrix placed at the repair results in regular dense collagen tissue with the use of our matrix plus our stem cells (Figs. 1.34 and 1.35).

The next question is what's going on mechanically? We found that our stem cell—seeded matrices allow for increased tendon biomechanics. With our control on the left, the group with the repair plus scaffold and cells, we found to have a significantly higher ultimate stress over the repair or the repair plus scaffold group (Fig. 1.36).

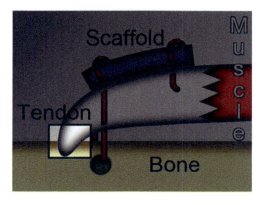

FIGURE 1.32 What is occurring at tendon insertion?

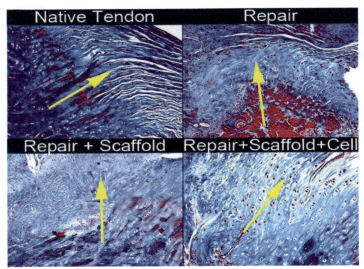

Arrow -direction of tendon-bone axis

FIGURE 1.33 What is occurring at tendon insertion? Cell seeding achieves insertion morphology similar to intact tendon. Cell-seeded scaffolds resulted in native-like tendon-bone insertion transition.

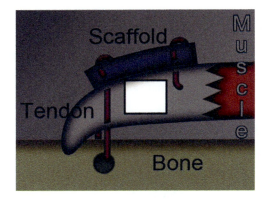

FIGURE 1.34 What is occurring at the tendon substance?

The use of our advanced materials in mesenchymal stem cell matrices for shoulder rotator cuff tendon regeneration allows for native tissue-like histology and greater tensile properties. When we went to look for the stem cells, we didn't find the stem cells in the area in the interior of the rotator cuff repair. What we think is happening is a paracrine effect that's taking place from the stem cells, where the cells are secreting trophic factors in the area. Also, we

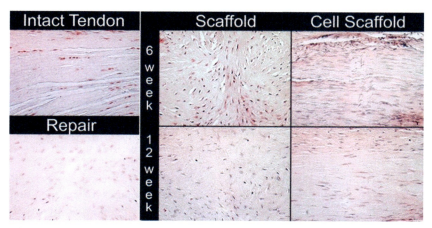

FIGURE 1.35 What is occurring at the tendon substance? Cell seeding accelerates tendon body remodeling. Cell seeding results in parallel organization of fibers with elongated cells underneath the scaffold.

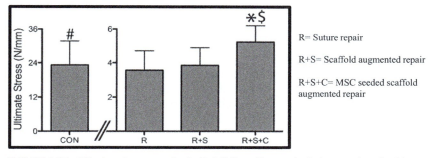

R= Suture repair

R+S= Scaffold augmented repair

R+S+C= MSC seeded scaffold augmented repair

FIGURE 1.36 What's going on mechanically? Cell seeding results in increased tendon biomechanics. At 6 and 12 weeks, MSC augmentation provides greater ultimate stress over repair and scaffold augmented repair.

believe there is an immunomodulatory effect taking place. The nanofiber matrices create a stem cell niche or environment that allows cells to be able to preserve their stem cell phenotype and to operate. We published this in the journal *Plos One*, Engineered Stem Cell Niche Matrices for Rotator Cuff Tendon and Regenerative Engineering.

It's also nice to see that the University has been very interested and involved in moving forward with our technologies. We hopefully will be able to bring this type of technology to people through clinical trials, soon.

So, what am I doing next? Well, this area of regenerative engineering is again the convergence of advanced material science, stem cell science, physics, developmental biology, and clinical translation for the regeneration of complex tissues, organs, and organ systems. We recently published a book called *Regenerative Engineering* that we've published in the area.

Sharing the Knowledge and Advancing the Field

We also have a new organization, the Regenerative Engineering Society, which is the first society for everyone, in that it democratizes and makes science available, affordable, and understandable to all (It's $20 for those individuals under age 20). This society is now a part of the American Institute of Chemical Engineers, as a community. And the website is located on the AICHE website.

We have a new journal called *Regenerative Engineering and Translational Medicine*, which we invite you to submit to. Every journal article has a lay summary. We also welcome laypeople to join and learn about the science involved in regenerative engineering.

We have an annual meeting called the Rockstars of Regenerative Engineering. This is where we bring three or four superstars of regeneration together for a day and a half program, where they are able to spend time with people and get together. Our latest Rockstars meeting was held last year in California. It's a large group, but not too large a group to be able to interact with individuals and to learn from. We are grateful to have major sponsorship from the National Science Foundation for these conferences.

This area of regenerative engineering is a convergence of these different fields. Since our very first paper in Science Translational Medicine, we've been able to move from there to books that continue to advance knowledge in the field. We've also had symposia on regenerative engineering, and it's great to see other individuals embrace the concepts and create symposia on their own.

Regenerative engineering centers are emerging across the country. One of the newest is the Center for Advanced Regenerative Engineering, CARE, at Northwestern University in Evanston, Illinois, which is doing great work.

At University of Connecticut, we're now trying to take what we're doing in the laboratory and move it forward in terms of clinical projects in patients.

So Much More on the Horizon

Well, what else is next? As amazing as it seems, we've now been able to regenerate pretty much every musculoskeletal tissue involved in the body, skin, nerve, ligaments, muscle, and bone. We're now dedicated to being able to really bring about and harness the principles of regeneration and work toward limb regeneration (Fig. 1.37).

Our big goal now is to regenerate lost limbs in humans, by the year 2030. We call this initiative the Hartford Engineering a Limb Project (HEAL). And we are proud of the work has been supported by the NIH Directors Pioneer Award.

Pushing the Limits of Science, Medicine, and Engineering

Our team has also been working on novel polyphosphazene-based materials. These are polymeric materials that are biocompatible and have neutral

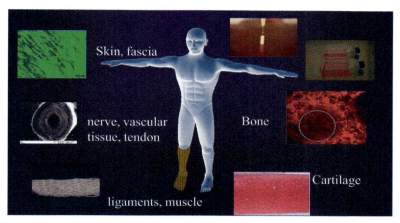

FIGURE 1.37 What is next? As amazing as it seems, we've now been able to regenerate pretty much every musculoskeletal tissue involved in the body, skin, nerve, ligaments, muscle, and bone. We're now dedicated to being able to really bring about and harness the principles of regeneration and work toward limb regeneration.

degradation products. It's a polymeric material, which will be extremely important for the future of tissue regeneration. They have design flexibility. They're more biocompatible than many traditional polymers. Our goal has been to develop mechanically competent polyphosphazene materials, blend it with traditional polylactic acid, glycolic acid materials, to utilize it to exploit a unique pore-forming ability that we've been able to find with these blends (Fig. 1.38).

The synthesis approach is a thermal ring opening polymerization to create this nitrogen—phosphorus backbone material. Then we can substitute side groups at the R1 and R2 position. We can blend them with polylactic acid and polyglycolic acid. We have found in a series of papers that by utilizing an amino acid side chain group, we can create materials that become miscible with polylactic acid—polyglycolic acid copolymers (Fig. 1.39).

That mechanism of miscibility is through hydrogen bonding between the polylactic acid, glycolic acid, and the amino acid peptide group of the poly-phosphazene material. We've utilized glycyl-glycine ethyl ester, which is a dipeptide that has a lot more hydrogen bonding and is biocompatible. Then we can also utilize a phenylalanine ethyl ester, which has an aryl group that brings about hydrophobic features. Our team has been able to use a phenyl-phenol, which has a high amount of hydrophobicity and can really help to modulate erosion. We can get some very, very interesting results in terms of the degradation characteristics that you'll see in terms of these materials (Figs. 1.40 and 1.41).

So "PY" is the material with the glycyl-glycine ethyl ester and the phenylalanine ethyl ester. And "PZ" is the glycyl-glycine ethyl ester

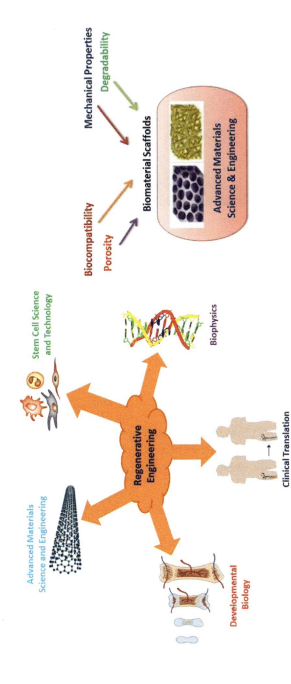

FIGURE 1.38 Regenerative engineering—advanced materials. Novel polyphosphazene-based biomaterials. *From Ogueri, K.S., Laurencin, C.T., 2020. Elsevier Encyclopedia of Bone Biology, 135-148; Ogueri, K.S., Allcock, H.R., Laurencin, C. T., 2019. Progress in Polymer Science 98, 101146.*

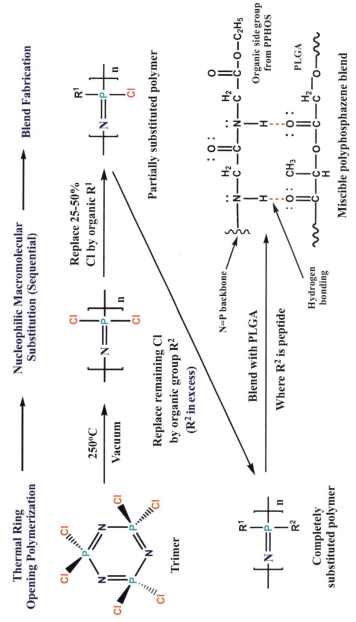

FIGURE 1.39 Regenerative engineering—advanced materials. Approach and theoretical framework.

Glycylglycine ethyl ester

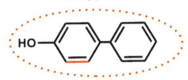

- Dipeptides impart more H bonding sites
- Biocompatible and biomimetic interactions

Phenylalanine ethyl ester

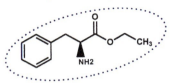

- Aryl group confer Hydrophobic features
- Biocompatible and hydrolytically active

Phenylphenol

- Its hydrophobicity utilized to modulate erosion
- Could affect physicochemical functions

FIGURE 1.40   Regenerative engineering—advanced materials. Side group selection.

containing material with the phenyl-phenol containing material. We can create both of them and blend them with our polylactic acid—glycolic acid copolymer. Again, using hydrogen bonding, we are able to create these different blend materials. Morphologically, it is due to the extensive hydrogen bonding of the polyphosphazenes, containing the amino acids on both of the R groups; we find small size domains and a well-distributed morphology (Fig. 1.42).

With our phenyl-phenol group, because of the great amount of hydrophobicity, we find that the presence of a dispersed phrase of PZ in the matrix. If we examine contact angle measurement, polylactic acid and glycolic acid are relatively hydrophilic. The polyphosphazenes with their hydrophobic side groups are relatively hydrophobic. As we blend them, we can modulate and control the hydrophobicity of the materials based upon our contact angle measurements as we see here (Fig. 1.43).

We can also get unique characteristics in terms of degradation. The blends themselves actually have degradation characteristics in terms of pH that are intermediate between polylactic acid and the polyphosphazenes. Polylactic acid, glycolic acid, and their copolymers are traditional polymers that are used in vivo in a number of different FDA-cleared devices. As you can see, we can create a material that modulates the pH into a more physiological range (Fig. 1.44).

What we also see is that with degradation of these different materials, the "PZ" containing the more hydrophobic phenyl-phenol side group can create a matrix that starts to form different types of microspheres. Whereas a "PY" does to a certain extent, the "PZ" does to a great extent.

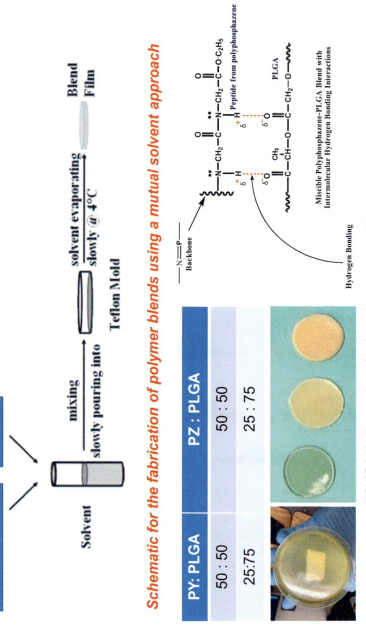

FIGURE 1.41   Regenerative engineering—advanced materials. Polymer blend fabrication.

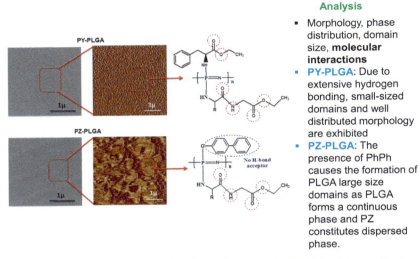

Analysis

- Morphology, phase distribution, domain size, **molecular interactions**
- **PY-PLGA**: Due to extensive hydrogen bonding, small-sized domains and well distributed morphology are exhibited
- **PZ-PLGA**: The presence of PhPh causes the formation of PLGA large size domains as PLGA forms a continuous phase and PZ constitutes dispersed phase.

FIGURE 1.42   Regenerative engineering—advanced materials. Molecular interactions.

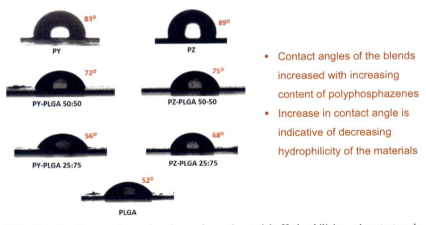

- Contact angles of the blends increased with increasing content of polyphosphazenes
- Increase in contact angle is indicative of decreasing hydrophilicity of the materials

FIGURE 1.43   Regenerative engineering—advanced materials. Hydrophilicity and contact angle.

We have examined this phenomenon using electrospray ionization mass spectrometry. We examined it after 12 weeks of degradation. What we find is that the peaks for the PZ component are very prominent after the blend degrades. The polylactic acid polyglycolic acid actually goes away. So, what we have shown is that the microspheres that are left after the degradation of the blend material are mainly this PZ material that's left afterward. We now have the prospect of being able to create a matrix where we place a block of polymer into a defect, and that block of polymer becomes a porous matrix over time (Fig. 1.45).

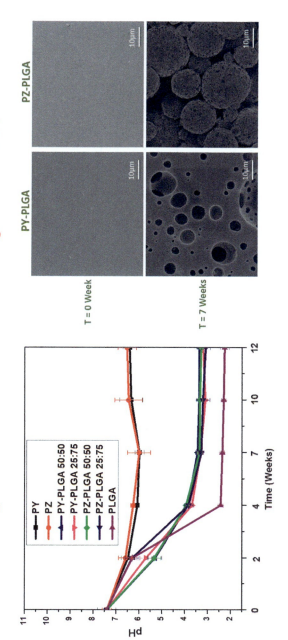

SEM images of the blends before and after degradation in PBS

- Blends generated degradation products with pH values higher than that of the PLGA
- Degradation products of PY and PZ constitute a natural buffer
- The new materials exhibited inherent pore-forming tendencies upon degradation

FIGURE 1.44 Regenerative engineering—advanced materials. Degradation study.

ESI-MS after 12-week Degradation

- ESI-MS signals with highest intensity are taken as 100% abundance
- Results confirmed that the microspheres after the degradation study were mainly composed of PZ polymers
- Peaks for PZ component were prominent before and after the blend degradation study
- PLGA peak disappeared after the PZ-PLGA blend underwent 12-week degradation.
- These results were similar to the ones for PY-PLGA

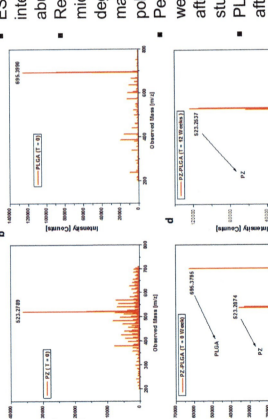

FIGURE 1.45 Regenerative engineering—advanced materials. Mechanistic study on erosion.

We've examined cell proliferation in these materials and have found that we get impressive cellular growth in vitro. We've placed these materials in an in vivo using an ulnar critical size defect model that we've discussed before (Fig. 1.46).

If we examine bone volume presence after 12 weeks in terms of these matrices, we can see higher bone volume in our blend matrices over the traditional polylactic acid—glycolic acid copolymer materials. With H&E and toluidine blue staining, we can find new bone and apposition to host bone that's there (Fig. 1.47).

The polyphosphazenes represent a class of extremely versatile polymers that we're now working with even more. It has a real prospect of being able to work on a number of regeneration type settings. The unique pore-forming ability of some of the polyphosphazene blends is particularly exciting.

We've been taking a new look at how we approach the regeneration of tissues, especially complex tissues. The work that we do in the field is usually a top-down approach, where we recreate biomimetics of tissues using matrices and try to have regeneration occur. In terms of limb generation, tissues are assembled from the cellular scale to produce intact structures (Fig. 1.3).

The blastema is a prime example. In terms of limb generation, a newt can regenerate a limb within 7—10 weeks. Of course, we're not newts. However, we believe that this must be part of the arsenal in terms of what we think about in regenerative engineering.

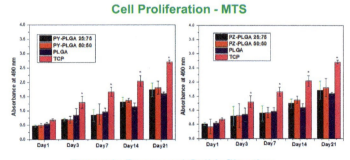

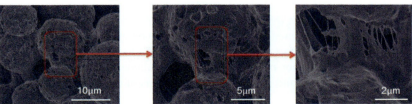

FIGURE 1.46   Regenerative engineering—advanced materials. In vitro osteocompatibility.

A.

Before & After Bone Defect PNGEGPhPh-PLGA Implantations

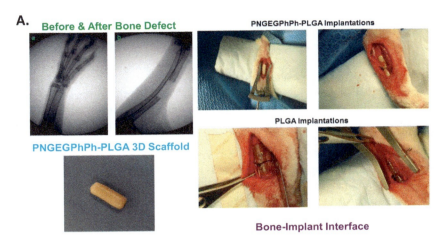

PNGEGPhPh-PLGA 3D Scaffold

PLGA Implantations

Bone-Implant Interface

FIGURE 1.47A Regenerative engineering—advanced materials. In vivo studies.

B.

Tissue Harvest and Isolation

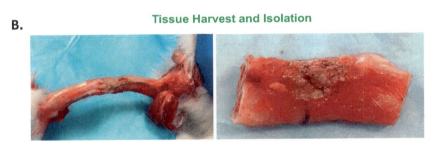

➢ Visual observation indicated no apparent inflammation or physical impairment

➢ No sign of systemic or neurological toxicity for the rabbits with both implants

➢ Harvested bone tissues for PNGEGPhPh-PLGA showed significant regeneration

➢ Early days of PLGA implantation showed mild inflammatory response – High rigidity

FIGURE 1.47B Regenerative engineering—advanced materials. In vivo studies.

Once while teaching surgical residents, I showed a picture of a finger of an individual that had been partially severed with a saw. While some might advocate amputation or a complicated surgical procedure, I asked what happens if we just treat it with dressing changes?

I showed them pictures after one week, and then after eight weeks. It had completely regenerated to their surprise. My lesson to them were that we can see that while we're not newts and we're not salamanders, we do have the ability to be newt-like and salamander-like in terms of our ability to be able to regenerate (Fig. 1.48).

C.

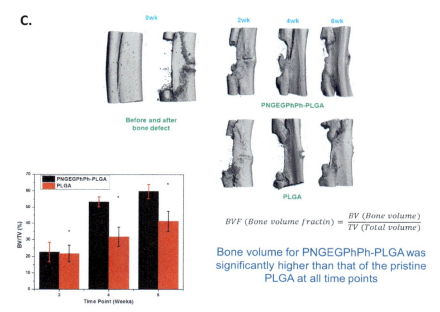

$$BVF\ (Bone\ volume\ fractin) = \frac{BV\ (Bone\ volume)}{TV\ (Total\ volume)}$$

Bone volume for PNGEGPhPh-PLGA was significantly higher than that of the pristine PLGA at all time points

FIGURE 1.47C   Regenerative engineering—advanced materials. In vivo studies, micro-CT analysis.

D.

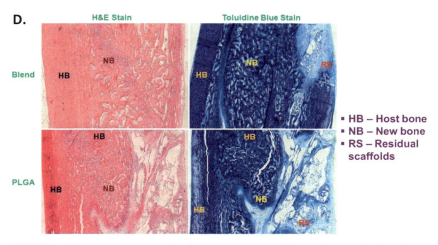

- HB – Host bone
- NB – New bone
- RS – Residual scaffolds

FIGURE 1.47D   Regenerative engineering—advanced materials. In vivo studies, histological analysis.

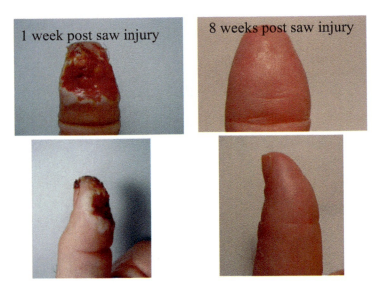

FIGURE 1.48 Nonoperative treatment healing.

Our new work is to try to harness the newt in us in terms of regeneration. We believe it will allow us to be able to move forward to find new ways to be able to regenerate tissues.

We're working in an area that we have termed "The Grid" as a novel tool for complex tissue regeneration in mammals. The story is that we know that humans have limited regenerative ability. But salamanders have extensive regenerative ability throughout their life span. We know that there are models for limb generation, such as the accessory limb model where a signal from a nerve is placed at a fracture site with opposing skin to allow for regeneration, and we can actually utilize that model to create extra limbs in salamanders (Fig. 1.4).

We know that limb generation is mediated by interactions between cells in salamanders. It has been hypothesized that there are pattern-forming cells that may be present providing positional information. In addition, there are pattern-following cells that help to remake the missing parts according to that positional information, which for example, includes stem cells (Fig. 1.49).

One of the things that our collaborator in this effort Dr. David Gardiner, Professor, Developmental & Cell Biology, School of Biological Sciences at the University of California, Irvine has done, is to make a limb from scratch with purified growth factors combined with purified heparin sulfate proteoglycan from a mammal using his accessory limb model. We were very, very fascinated with this ability to be able to create a limb in a salamander from scratch, a separate limb, utilizing heparin sulfate proteoglycan. We started to examine heparin sulfate as a material that might be able to help us in terms of the

Which Cells Possess Positional Information?

> ➤ Limb regeneration is mediated by interactions between cells
> > ❖ Pattern forming cells provide positional information
> > ❖ Pattern following cells remake the missing parts according to positional information (e.g. progenitor cells, adult stem cells)

> ➤ The signaling mechanism for pattern formation are less understood.

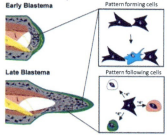

FIGURE 1.49   There are pattern-following cells that help to remake the missing parts according to that positional information, which, for example, includes stem cells. *From McCusker, C., Bryant, S.V., Gardiner, D.M., 2015. Regeneration 2(2):54-71.*

> ➤ Heparan sulfate (HS) can bind to lots of morphogens and cytokines to mediate these signaling pathways e.g. FGFs, BMPs, Wnts, shh

> ➤ HS is a glycosaminoglycan (GAG) chain located cell surface and extra cellular matrix (ECM)

> ➤ HS can induce ectopic pattern formation in axolotl limb.

> ➤ Some sulfotransferases are differentially expressed in blastema

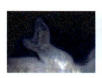 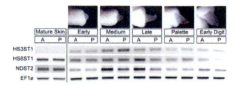

This project focused on the presence of pattern forming cells in limb.

FIGURE 1.50   Heparan sulfate (HS) may hold a key to control pattern formation. *From Phan, A.Q., Lee, J., Oei, M., et al. 2015. Regeneration, 182-201.*

regeneration process. We found that there are various heparin sulfates that are actually produced during the time of limb regeneration (Fig. 1.50).

We began examining cells in the axolotl salamander. And we found heparin sulfate-rich cells that possess these multiple branching cell processes. We've termed these cells as positional information cells. And we've called them grid cells. We call them grid because these are groups that are regenerative, dispersed, and dendritic. We recently published the first paper on them (Figs. 1.51 and 1.52).

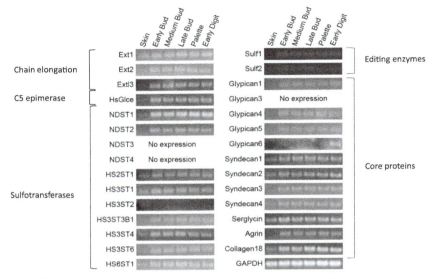

FIGURE 1.51 Various HS-related genes upregulation during limb regeneration. *From Otsuka, T., Phan, A.Q., Laurencin, C.T., Esko, J.D., Bryant, S.V., Gardiner, D.M., 2020. Regenerative Engineering and Translational Medicine 6(1):7-17.*

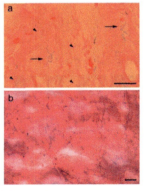

- HS-rich cells possessed multiple branching cell processes
- These cells were arranged in a grid and their multiple cellular processes overlapped with processes.
- We termed these cells as positional information GRID (Groups that are Regenerative, Interspersed and Dendritic) cells

FIGURE 1.52 Identification of pattern forming HS-rich cells in axolotl dermis. *From Otsuka, T., Phan, A.Q., Laurencin, C.T., Esko, J.D., Bryant, S.V., Gardiner, D.M., 2020. Regenerative Engineering and Translational Medicine 6(1):7-17.*

We found these grid cells were localized in the connective tissues (Fig. 1.53).

They were associated with differentiated tissues of the limb. At a later stage of blastema formation, we have found these grid cells appeared (Fig. 1.54).

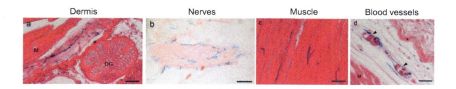

GRID cells were localized in the connective tissues
associated with the differentiated tissues of the limb.

FIGURE 1.53   Grid cells localization within the connective tissues in the limb. *From Otsuka, T.,
Phan, A.Q., Laurencin, C.T., Esko, J.D., Bryant, S.V., Gardiner, D.M., 2020. Regenerative Engineering and Translational Medicine 6(1):7-17.*

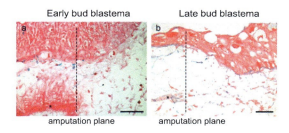

- GRID cells were not evident at the early stage of blastema
  formation distal to the amputationplane.
- At later stage of blastema, GRID cells reappeared distal to
  the amputation plane, but not distaltip.

FIGURE 1.54   The distribution of GRID cells during regeneration. *From Otsuka, T., Phan, A.Q.,
Laurencin, C.T., Esko, J.D., Bryant, S.V., Gardiner, D.M., 2020. Regenerative Engineering and
Translational Medicine 6(1):7-17.*

Then they reappeared distal to the amputation point. What is exciting is
that we've also identified these similar grid cells in mouse limb skin. This
presents the possibility of these cells being found in all mammals (Fig. 1.55).

Grid cells are candidates for these pattern-forming cells, as we've called
them, to allow for the pattern following cells to be able to better foster
complex regeneration. They hold great potential in our eyes to provide the
positional information that may enhance regeneration in humans. So we're
actively working in this exciting area.

The other area of our new work is on advanced biologics. We are focused
on the use of amnion as an advanced biologic for tissue regeneration. Our
ultimate goal is limb regeneration, and we think that a holistic unsiloed
approach is necessary to achieve this (Fig. 1.56).

In the past work on regeneration, chemists, surgeons, and engineers have
all worked separately on their pieces of the puzzle. It is time for a big paradigm shift—a transdisciplinary approach that melds the cutting-edge technologies from all the sciences—physical, chemical, biology, material, and

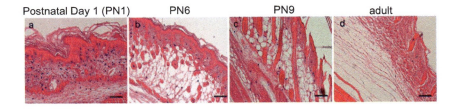

Postnatal Day 1 (PN1) PN6 PN9 adult

- GRID cells were also identified in mouse limbskin.
- The abundance of GRID cells changeontogenetically.

FIGURE 1.55 Abundance of mammalian grid cells in neonatal mice skin. *From Otsuka, T., Phan, A.Q., Laurencin, C.T., Esko, J.D., Bryant, S.V., Gardiner, D.M., 2020. Regenerative Engineering and Translational Medicine 6(1):7-17.*

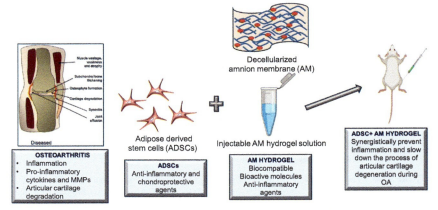

FIGURE 1.56 Amnion as an advanced biologic for tissue regeneration. Develop amnion-based hydrogel as delivery system for adipose-derived stem cells for osteoarthritis treatment.

engineering sciences along with cutting-edge stem cell research, physics, and clinical translation for the regeneration of complex tissues and organ systems.

As the only surgeon who has ever been inducted into the Academies of Science, Medicine, and Innovation, I continue to push for deconstructing the walls that slow down our progress. And we must remember that at the heart of all this progress is clinician participation. We must continue to gain deeper understandings of the body's capabilities to regenerate. I know that when I am doing a surgical procedure to repair a tear, I am counting on the body to do its part to heal and regenerate tissue. So, as we bring together all the research and science of regeneration, we must always look to what the body can do to regenerate itself as a major piece of the puzzle.

Our team is very interested in the treatment of osteoarthritis on the road to limb generation (Fig. 1.57).

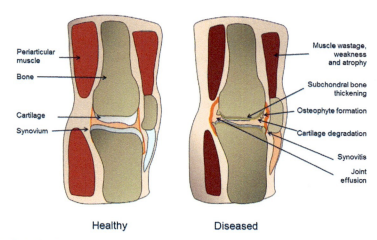

FIGURE 1.57   Amnion as an advanced biologic for tissue regeneration. Background: osteoarthritis (OA). *From Johnson, C.I., Argyle, D.J., Clements, D.N., 2016. The Veterinary Journal 209, 40-49.*

There are systems for adipose-derived stem cell therapy that have been suggested for the treatment of osteoarthritis. Adipose-derived stem cells have both antiinflammatory effects and also chondroprotective effects that we know, but without a material delivery system, there could be inadequate cellular distribution and inadequate cellular survival, and poor stem cell retention (Fig. 1.58).

It would be desirable to have an ideal carrier matrix system to create an optimized delivery system.

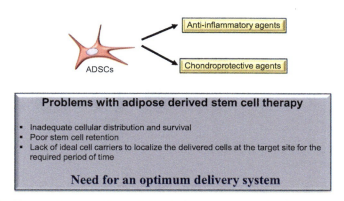

FIGURE 1.58   Amnion as an advanced biologic for tissue regeneration. Background: Adipose-derived stem cells (ADSCs) for OA.

The Power and Potential of Amnion

We've worked with injectable amnion. It's a material that on its own is anti-inflammatory and antibacterial and suppresses proinflammatory cytokines. Our goal was to create a system where we could combine both amnion- and adipose-derived stem cells to allow for regeneration.

We created an amnion hydrogel using a decellularization process followed by lyophilization, and an enzymatic digested step. We can create a substance that gels at physiological pH and temperature and that at room temperature is a liquid (Fig. 1.59).

A.

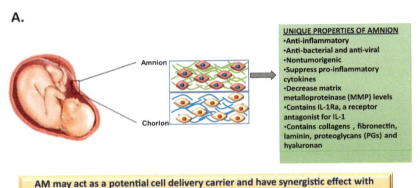

UNIQUE PROPERTIES OF AMNION
•Anti-inflammatory
•Anti-bacterial and anti-viral
•Nontumorigenic
•Suppress pro-inflammatory cytokines
•Decrease matrix metalloproteinase (MMP) levels
•Contains IL-1Ra, a receptor antagonist for IL-1
•Contains collagens , fibronectin, laminin, proteoglycans (PGs) and hyaluronan

AM may act as a potential cell delivery carrier and have synergistic effect with ADSCs in reducing inflammation and cartilage degradation in OA.

FIGURE 1.59A Background: amnion membrane (AM) injectable hydrogel.

B.

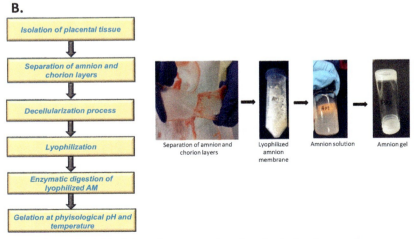

FIGURE 1.59B Schematic representation of amnion hydrogel preparation.

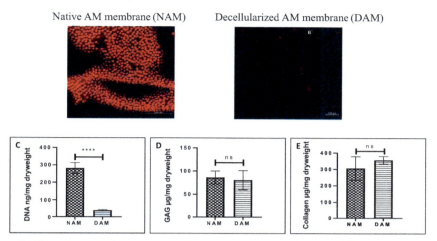

FIGURE 1.60   Decellularization of amnion membrane and quantification of ECM components.

We have quantified the components of the gel and demonstrated that we've been able to decellularize it (Fig. 1.60).

We could do basic engineering in terms of modulating the shear rate and shear stress of the gel based upon the concentration of the amnion material in the solution. We have seeded cells, adipose-derived stem cells. We've studied cell growth and viability and their dependence upon the density and shear stress of the amnion gel. We've also studied the stemness of these cells seeded onto the gel and confirmed that amnion gel can allow cells to maintain their stem cell characteristics (Fig. 1.61).

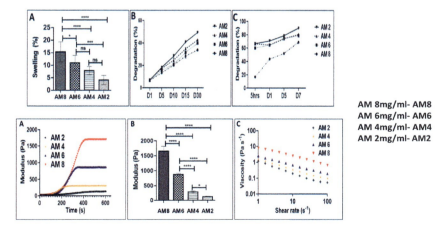

FIGURE 1.61   Amnion hydrogel characterization.

Next, we began to examine the effects of the amnion, adipose-derived stem cells, and the combination of amniotic and adipose-derived stem cells. We create a model where we treated chondrocytes with IL-1beta and then further treated alone or with adipose-derived stem cells or with amnion or a combination of an adipose-derived stem cells and amnion. What we can see is that with all treatment groups, we find effects on levels of MMP, MMP13, IL-6, and TIMP. The use of the combination of adipose-derived stem cells and amnion in vitro appears to have a synergistic effect in terms of its effects on levels of cytokines (Fig. 1.62).

Then we created an osteoarthritis model in the rat where we utilize the collagenase injection to induce osteoarthritis (Fig. 1.63).

We have four groups. Our control, an adipose-derived stem cell–treated group, an amnion hydrogel-treated group, and amnion hydrogel and adipose-derived stem cell combined treatment group. Our research has shown that we can compare our collagenase-injected osteoarthritis histology to our sham surgery histology. Compared with A, B shows marked synovitis and also erosions denoted by the loss of Safranin-O staining (Fig. 1.64).

After induction of osteoarthritis and treatment, we find that with the phosphate-buffered saline control, again, we have continuous synovitis that's present. We really have almost a pristine area with the amnion hydrogel and our adipose-derived stem cells combined. If we examine our histology with our control after collagenase injection, we have loss of Safranin-O staining with erosions that are present (Fig. 1.65).

Our adipose-derived stem cell treatment group still shows a significant amount of erosions, with some improvement. And the amnion hydrogel has an even more improved response. The amnion hydrogel plus adipose-derived stem cells provided a synergistically positive response in terms of the return of the safranin-O staining in cartilage.

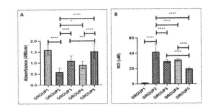

Group **1**: Untreated chondrocytes, Group **2**: Chondrocytes treated with 20 ng/mL IL-1β, Group **3**: Chondrocytes with IL-1β (20 ng/mL) and ADSCs, Group **4**: Chondrocytes with IL-1β (20 ng/mL), and AM (6mg/ml) and, Group **5**: Chondrocytes with IL-1β (20 ng/mL) and ADSCs encapsulated within AM

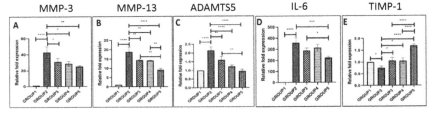

FIGURE 1.62 Antiinflammatory and chondroprotective effects of ADSCs and AM.

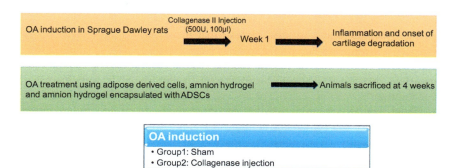

FIGURE 1.63 Intraarticular injection of ADSCs in amnion hydrogel in OA rat model.

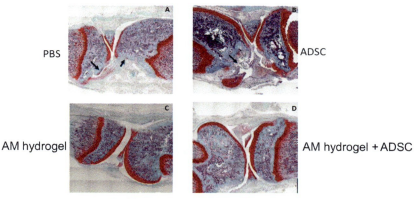

FIGURE 1.64 OA treatment: safranin-0 staining.

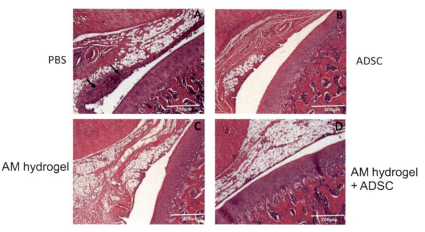

FIGURE 1.65 OA treatment: hematoxylin and eosin staining.

We believe that our amnion hydrogel is a promising carrier for adipose-derived stem cells, and we also believe that these can act synergistically to exert an antiinflammatory and confer protective effect. We are continuing to study this combination in larger animals. We believe that this may be an important alternative treatment for osteoarthritis and for use in complex tissue regeneration.

These new technologies will be important to the Hartford Engineering a Limb Project. I still remember coming to Beijing when I was elected to the Chinese Academy of Engineering when I first announced it. My speech appeared in China News Daily. I was later told that the headline on the article translated to Regenerative Engineering Moonshot, and it is a moonshot. But the last time I checked, we did make it to the moon.

I look forward to continuing our work in complex tissue regeneration. It is a multiyear, multidimensional quest not only for limb regeneration but also for the clinical treatment of a number of musculoskeletal diseases.

It Takes a Talented Team to Pull Off a Moonshot

I have been blessed to be surrounded by a talented team of students and researchers who dare to dream, think, and be persistent. For every brick wall we hit in research together, we work to find a new window. My success in this field is due really from their success.

This kind of research and the results that come from it are only made possible through the support of funders. My research has been funded by the National Institute of Health since 1982. The National Science Foundation, the Department of Defense, and also the NIH Director's Pioneer Award have been integral partners in funding our limb regeneration work over the years.

At this stage of my career, so much of it feels like full circle moments. I began working on these things in a start-up lab at MIT while I was doing my residency across the river at Massachusetts General Hospital. With no money for lab assistants, I got help from volunteer undergraduate science and engineering majors. Aside from those bright undergraduates, I was on my own. Six years later I moved my laboratory from MIT to Drexel University in Philadelphia. One postdoctoral fellow came with me.

Some years later, I moved to the University of Virginia. By then, my laboratory had grown, and ten other researchers moved along with me. Five years later, we all came to the University of Connecticut, but now there were 14 of us.

Now the team that's around me works on our projects at the Connecticut Convergence Institute for Translation in Regenerative Engineering. We've become more than a department or an institute, in important ways we've become a community. In particular, over the years I've come to develop and share certain principles. Most of these principles have come from my own life experiences. Some have been imbued in me by my mentors and teachers, and I have tried hard to pass them on. All of them shape my life as a surgeon, engineer, and someone deeply involved in issues of social justice.

Diversity, Social Justice, Equity, and Me

I have always worked at the interface of medicine and engineering and am also someone who is very much involved in issues of social justice. It is not enough for me to be working at the top of my game; it is important that we create opportunities to expose our young Black and Brown people to the sciences and to STEM. Our Institute is working to open the pipeline and prepare them to work to be the best in medicine, engineering, and research. It is an important mission, and I will discuss this more later in the book.

I was very excited and very proud to receive the Herbert Nickens Award. It's the American Association of Medical Colleges' highest award for social justice and equity, and it recognizes the work that I have been involved in over the past almost 40 years in the area of social justice and equity.

It reflects my values and efforts to create a fairer society for all in work that has ranged from boots on the ground programs seeking to increase the numbers of Black and Brown people working in engineering, science, and medicine, to larger programs such as the creation of The W. Montague Cobb National Medical Association Institute program looking at ways in which one can address disparities in health, medicine, and science for Black people, to launching a new journal—the Journal of Racial and Ethnic Health Disparities—which is now the leading journal working in the space, to our new work in terms of Chairing the National Academy of Sciences, Engineering and Medicine Roundtable on Black Men and Black Women in Science, Engineering and Medicine, and the recent Spingard Medal from the NAACP.

Our main challenge in terms of equity for Black people in both the United States and the world is the persistence of racism. We know that there are excess deaths each year of Black people linked to racism and we have known this for a very, very long time—this is not new news. In the 1990s, the National Medical Association had a consensus report examining racism and its effects on health and the creation of health disparities. The National Academies followed up with a study called "Unequal Treatment," which examined the unequal treatment of Black people and others in the United States and found racism to be a primary reason why this is happening.

In 2020 we saw the murders of George Floyd and Breonna Taylor garner widespread media attention. This injustice translates to the medical establishment, too, in terms of medical care, which translates to higher mortality for Black people. That is the major challenge we have to address in terms of healthcare and something that I am very passionate about.

We recently made the case for why we need to see more Black professionals working in medicine, along with science and engineering. On the medical side, Black physicians treating Black patients obviously do not exhibit the levels of unconscious bias and conscious racism that take place among white physicians and some new studies—for example, in COVID-19—have suggested that clinical outcomes are improved where Black physicians have taken care of Black patients.

Number one is that there are so many systemic racism issues. That we still must address. It was extreme when I was coming up—I still remember walking into a classroom at MIT and having a professor physically block me from coming into the door. Is it still this extreme? Probably not as blatant, but just as damaging. The ultimate goal of the Hartford Engineering A Limb (HEAL) project, under active research in my laboratory, is aimed at helping wounded warriors as well as others who have lost limbs or experienced joint damage. Other patients who could benefit from the future breakthroughs are those with amputations due to bone cancer, diabetes, dangerous infections, or trauma accidents, or even children born with missing or impaired limbs.

I was very fortunate to win the Presidential Award for Excellence in Science, Math, and Engineering mentorship from President Obama and the American Association for Advancement of Science Mentor Award, so mentoring is a big component of my life.

I think for mentors it is important that there is a dedication to that individual and to their long-term future. I have been fortunate to have mentorships that have been lifelong; I am still in contact with people I have mentored who are now full professors and chairs or deans. I think it is also important that the mentorship is a two-way relationship—meaning that there are expectations from both the mentor and the mentee. The mentees have to follow up with and listen to their mentors. It is not necessarily that the person has to agree with what their mentor says, but there has to be a clear relationship in which the counsel or guidance is provided and has been well thought through. Finally, there has got to be an open dialogue about successes, setbacks, and plans.

Yes, I think you do need to have a representative workforce to be able to have equity in medicine, for a number of reasons. Number one—because, as we alluded to, when you have Black and Brown physicians, you reduce the levels of unconscious bias and racism in the system as a whole and that results in better quality of care. Number two is that to a great extent the underrepresentation of Black physicians in medicine right now is a symptom of a system that has at its roots systemic racism.

One marker for how we progress is to examine the numbers of Black people who are in medical school. We had a historic low in terms of Black men in medicine around 2014—15. Those numbers have rebounded a bit, but that shows that even in a world in which we talk about diversity and equity, such a phenomenon can happen. That's why I published my piece "The Context of Diversity" in the journal Science. You cannot think of diversity as an old

Kumbaya general feeling. We have to look at what's happening with specific groups and with the specific challenges that are taking place in specific groups. With Black people, especially in the United States, we know that racism plays a role in every aspect of their life.

I also wrote a paper recently on racial profiling, as a public health issue, speaking to how racial profiling by police in America has serious health effects. This is an area that really needs to be addressed.

In the "Healthcare Hero" article I wrote, I discussed how and why the coronavirus was and still is disproportionally affecting Blacks. I recall that when Covid-19 first hit, there was a myth of Black immunity that was circulating on the Internet and social media, so I set out to examine that because I was really concerned if that misinformation got out, it could be disastrous for the Black community.

I published the first peer-reviewed study in the nation with these findings in April. It exploded the myth and created an early warning that the disease could be particularly bad for the Black community.

It's important to understand that the reason the levels that we're seeing are this high is because of the history of discrimination that has taken place in this country.

When thinking about remedies for the issue at hand, I developed the concept of the IDEAL Pathway to creating a just and equitable society. Currently, we're in a world of discussions about diversity, inclusion, and equity. While we have had some gains in these areas, they have not really sufficiently addressed the issues of racism that we see in this country. So, my belief is that we need to move to inclusion, diversity, equity, antiracism, and learning (IDEAL). Understanding ways in which Black people are affected by the specific kinds of racial discrimination called anti-Blackness. Understanding the history of Black, Indigenous, and all people of color. Moving from ally to what I would call a ride-or-die partner in the antiracism movement—these are some of the ways that I believe learning can be used in a constructive way to bring about the ideal pathway to move forward.

The proud moments are too numerous to count. I am blessed and highly favored. The moments surrounding my family (meeting and falling in love with my wife, and the birth of my children probably count as the best moments).

For me, starting the new field of regenerative engineering, taking care of patients as a surgeon, working for social justice, and mentoring the next generation, all while doing the most important thing: staying connected to my family, my values, and my God—collectively represent my purpose.

A life on purpose is where I am, which is the ultimate goal.

This book is about principles for success in this field and in life. They've served to guide my success in science and medicine, and in the businesses that have spun off from our developments. They have to do with leadership, with mentoring, with taking risks, and with how to realize your full potential, not just in the things you do, but in the business of living the fullest life possible.

I think of them as rules for personal achievement. But, of course, personal achievement is never just personal. "Life and leadership can't be about *me*," as Colin Powell has so wisely put it, "they have to be about *us*." The most valuable lessons I've learned have come from mentors who taught this truth side by side with truths about discovery and creativity.

My greatest good fortune was to have had the friendship and guidance of people who have inspired whole fields of endeavor in science and medicine: People like Judah Folkman, "the smartest man at Harvard," whose humility and compassion were legendary; Robert Langer, who turned a degree in chemical engineering into a career as a healer (and who was, not so coincidentally, Judah Folkman's protégé); and Leon Eisenberg, the preeminent psychiatrist who melded medical science and humanism and trained people like Paul Farmer and Jim Kim.

Great investigators and scientists that they were (are still, in Langer's case), each of them answered what Dr. Martin Luther King Jr. called "Life's most persistent and urgent question: What are you doing for others?" They taught by their example that the complete life is not just the life of achievement in whatever field your talents lie. It is also a life that seeks the wholeness of the giving and committed spirit.

And while my career has been filled with focus and planning, let me tell you about a time when it was actually pretty cool to be me. In 1996, I was in Holland to make a speech and went to the hotel bar. I was the only person of color there. Then I noticed several Black men come in for a drink too. They looked familiar, and then it hit me who they were—Earth Wind and Fire. What are the odds that I would meet them in Holland. I am and have always been a big fan of them and their music. We started talking, and I was trying to be cool. I said something like, "I respect your work." Ok, who says that to Earth, Wind, and Fire? And that's exactly how they looked at me. After all they are arguably one of the best bands of all time. I noticed that one of the members of the group was missing. When I asked about it, they told me that he had dislocated his shoulder and was up in his room. Well, I asked to see him. After all, injuries like this are a part of my specialty, as an orthopaedic surgeon and sports medicine doctor. They didn't get it at first, but I finally explained that I am the shoulder guy. And that's what we did. When next we met, they called me when they were in Philly to do a show. They invited my wife and I to come backstage. And we had a great time. But their next stop was scheduled for New York City on September 11, 2001. All events in New York had been canceled and they were stranded in Philly for 4 days. We invited them over, and we ended up jamming in our living room. Let me say it again. Earth, Wind, and Fire played in our living room.

Chapter 2

The Basics

Much of my career has been in science, and I will expand upon some of the work I presented in the first chapter.

But first, I have to take a moment to discuss the great UConn Huskies basketball program. As sports medicine and shoulder doctor, I have, of course been a great sports fan. My favorite professional team is the Philadelphia 76ers. I've been a season ticket holder for over 25 years, a dream for someone who grew up in the inner city of Philadelphia. I've had the opportunity to meet many of the great 76ers including Allen Iverson, someone I've followed through his triumphs, opportunities, challenges, trials, and tragedies. I admire him.

But back to the UConn Huskies. Collectively, the women's and men's basketball programs represent the greatest combination dynasty in college basketball. I've been fortunate to have been present for magnificent runs of achievement by both teams and have received the "bling" on the way.

An important point I want to make at the outset is that life is very short. Find things that you are passionate about and that you identify to be fun. Pursue your passion whether it be sports, or anything else. Success in life without enjoyment of life is not success at all.

In the first section, I told you a lot about what I do as an orthopaedic surgeon and sports medicine doctor. I shared my academic journey from getting a chemical engineering degree from Princeton to Harvard Medical School and the twists and turns of meshing science, research, medicine, and engineering to move regenerative engineering to the forefront of breakthrough science, and what it took for me to get it.

But who is Cato T. Laurencin? When you talk about my successes in life, you have to look at the way I define myself. I am so much more than the work and the accolades that you may see.

I am a family man, a husband, and a father. Family is very important to me. It's always a work of progress, and along with my relationship with God, it is the most important thing in my life. My wife graduated in Science from Hampton University, taught school for a time, and then made the decision to raise and take care of our children full-time. Our children are our joy. Not only are they smart and beautiful, but they also each exhibit a unique sense of humanity that makes them individually special and complex.

Success Is What You Leave Behind. https://doi.org/10.1016/B978-0-12-417224-1.00002-X
65

My schedule as an engineer, surgeon, and scientist can often be hectic. I also spent a great deal of time speaking around the world, giving lectures, providing demonstrations, and eventually even winning awards.

I was fortunate at a very early age in my career to meet Professor Hari Reddi. Dr. Reddi is one of the fathers of bone morphogenetic protein and was someone that I looked up to a lot as a scientist. As great as he is as a scientist, he is a superbly great person. He exudes warmth and compassion.

Anyway, I remember attending one of my first scientific meetings after I became a member of the faculty of Allegheny University and Drexel University in Philadelphia. There was Dr. Reddi, who provided his typical warm welcome to me. At his side, was his son. I was struck by this. I thought it was so wonderful that he had brought his son to the scientific meeting. It also presented an "aha" moment for me. His son was not only experiencing the science presented in the meeting, but he was also bonding with his father. I took that thought and that moment with me.

Fast forward a few years. I was at home in our living room in Philadelphia with my three children, and I announced that I was going to a scientific meeting in Italy.

Looking at me wide-eyed, my children asked how long I would be gone. I remarked that it would be a quick meeting and that it would take me 2 days. All the kids expressed clear sadness, and said "Dad, can you stay away longer?"

My children wanted to invoke the three-day rule. If I went to a scientific meeting internationally that lasted 3 days or more, I would take a child with me. "I guess I can stretch the meeting to 3 days." I said in response to their question.

By that point, the kids had already come up with a schedule regarding who was next to travel with me.

The international experiences with my individual children were so incredibly important. First, my kids were exposed to a broad array of science during our travels. It's no wonder that all of my children are scientists or engineers. Second, my children had the opportunity of meeting some of the greatest scientists/humanists in the world. The following picture is of my daughter Victoria in Italy at the World Academy of Sciences meeting. She is with Professor C.N.R. Rao, India's greatest scientist.

Not only is Professor Rao a splendid scientist, but he is also a writer of children's books. I was so grateful and pleased to see one of his children's books waiting for us on our return from Italy with a special inscription to my daughter in its pages.

The experience of traveling across the world one-on-one with your children is truly once in a lifetime and unforgettable. I count them as some of the most enjoyable times of my life. In addition, the bonding experience, I believe, is responsible for much of the cohesion in our family. I am so proud of my children, and that pride really grew, seeing them grow on the international stage.

While the international stage was transformative, I think for my children, the national stage was important, too. And so, I soon began to look for opportunities to bring my children to meetings where I could. I remember "take your daughter to work day" specifically. I was a member of the Advisory Committee on Engineering at the National Science Foundation and asked if I could bring my middle daughter to the all-day meeting. The staff persons were delighted to have her come and were very gracious in accommodating her. I still remember entering an expansive (and intimidating) board room in which the 18 or so members sat around the table. There, next to me was a name card for my daughter (an honorary committee member!) with her seat at the table.

Two things struck me particularly about that day. The first was the impact of mentorship. Professor Bill Wulf of the University of Virginia who served as President of the National Academy of Engineering was in attendance and spent a good time speaking with my daughter. Professor Wulf had previously been a professor at Carnegie Mellon University and is a world expert in computer sciences. If we fast-forward, my daughter attended Carnegie Mellon University, completed her bachelor's and master's in electrical engineering with work in computer sciences, and now works for a computer sciences company. I believe the early exposure and mentoring by Bill Wulf at that meeting had a huge effect.

The second thing that struck me (and please forgive a father's pride) was how supersmart and fearless my daughter was. At the meeting of the advisory committee that day, an agenda item was on improving engagement with younger people in engineering. The debate went on regarding strategies to recruit and retain engineers and how to build interest in engineering. One person on the committee asked, "Are we really special … is that the reason why we are not attracting more young people to engineering?"

At that point someone on the committee said, "well we have a young person here at table, why don't we consult with her." Some bristled and even were unhappy that my daughter might be placed in an embarrassing position. She was there for "take your daughter to work day" and not as a consultant. My daughter then surprised them all. Rather than responding to the question, she lithely left her seat and walked slowly and deliberately to the podium in the front of the room. She proceeded then in initiating a vigorous dialogue with members of the committee based on the central tenet of engineering: translating science to humanity.

I am so proud of all three of my children.

Another important facet of my life is that of working for justice and social change. I'm not quite sure when the sense of purpose in this was imbued in me. Perhaps it is in a name. My grandmother was Madge McIntosh Moorehead, and she was born near the turn of the 19th century. She was an important link to our past in many ways. She made it a point to tell me to always remember the origin of my name Cato. A family contemporary of hers was Dr. Cato Wilson, class of 1895 of Meharry Medical College. He was the immediate inspiration for my name by my parents, and an inspiration for my mother to attend Meharry Medical College and become a doctor.

But according to my grandmother, the Cato name stretched into the 1800s in Georgia and the 1700s in South Carolina.

I have pursued my grandmother's contention that our name Cato can be found over the past four centuries. Our family graveyard Georgia contains the gravesite of another Cato Wilson. A forebear of Dr. Cato Wilson, his gravestone states he was born in 1811. A visit to Charleston, South Carolina, for a scientific meeting led me to meet with historians and explore my grandmother's stories of a person named Cato who led a slave rebellion in the south.

This led me to the site of the Stono Rebellion, also known as Cato's Rebellion. I believe this was the Cato my grandmother referred to. She made it clear to me that I had a duty to help make things right in the world and live up to the name.

My parents were also important factors I think in my pursuit of justice and fairness. My father was originally born in St. Lucia. He was an incredible carpenter and was a staunch supporter of his beloved Carpenters' Union. I believe his devotion to the union came from his embracing the principles behind it, those being, the right of workers to organize and join a union that can negotiate with employers for a decent contract, a fair day's work for a fair day's pay, decent retirement and health benefits, safety on the job, top-level training and skills and perhaps most importantly, dedication to helping one another and the community. His rule was the union's rule, which was the Golden Rule: "Do unto others as you would have them do unto you." He was passionate and had an uncompromising will to succeed. I see that in myself.

My mother was born in Philadelphia. She taught in the segregated South and went to medical school in the same segregated South. She had planned to take those skills back to Philadelphia to open a private practice medical office. My mother was one of very few Black women to practice medicine in Philadelphia back when she began. Her practice. She was devoted to North Philadelphia. With numerous opportunities to move to more affluent parts of the city or suburbs, she lived and worked in North Philadelphia for 45 years. That's the pursuit of social justice.

My mother was unafraid. A case in point involved a march I believe in the 1970s led by the Reverend Jesse Jackson in Philadelphia. My mother took her young children by the hand and marched, too. It was there that I really appreciated the work, intelligence, and insight that Reverend Jesse Jackson has.

As the march was to begin, Reverend Jackson announced that this would be a peaceful march, with an emphasis on peace. We all nodded our heads, of course, in agreement. After about 15 minutes of marching, Reverend Jackson stopped and addressed the crowd again, emphasizing that this was a peaceful march. At that point, many of us just stated "of course" and didn't understand why the point was reiterated. Interestingly, at that point, my mother just told us to "stay close" with a calm and reassuring look.

About 15 minutes later, as we marched, we were slowly surrounded by a new police presence. Minutes later a small but vocal group of marchers pulled out banners and started chanting "They Killed Our King in '68, What Do We Have to Celebrate." Then I realized why Reverend Jackson had reiterated that the march was to be peaceful. As police began moving toward us, I saw Reverend Jackson deftly give a nod. The small but vocal group was cordoned off, and the march proceeded peacefully. I've always remembered my mother's look to me that day. It's the look and demeanor I try to emulate when the pressure is on.

My early experiences with each of my parents shaped my views regarding racial and social justice, fairness, and equity. Other experiences in the third part of the book have also been important in that regard. My work now is at the local, regional, and national levels and has shaped who I am and vice versa.

A significant part of my professional and personal life has revolved around my involvement with the National Medical Association. My earliest memories of the National Medical Association involve my mother and her love for the organization. Many may have forgotten, but the racist practices of the American Medical Association (AMA) precluded Blacks from becoming members even when I was growing up. When the AMA finally allowed Blacks to be members of the organization, they for years created and upheld requirements for county members to become national members. If counties continued to discriminate and not allow Blacks to become members, they could not become national members. This was significant because issues such as other organizational memberships, memberships on hospital clinical staffs etc. sometimes hinged on having membership in the AMA which whites easily had.

The National Medical Association (NMA) was started in 1895 and among its founders were some of the finest physicians in the country. A cornerstone of the NMA has been education. It runs the most comprehensive medical education scientific assembly I have ever seen. Among its leadership ranks during the era of my mother's involvement were senior medical leaders from the historically Black medical schools and other leading physicians in the country. The tradition continues.

The NMA membership includes a veritable who's who among Blacks in medicine. The NMA also encourages like-minded of any race and ethnicity to join.

My involvement with the NMA began just after completing my MD at the Harvard Medical School and my PhD at MIT. I started on my unique opportunity, to join the faculty of MIT as an Instructor of Biochemical Engineering, while starting a residency in orthopaedic surgery at Harvard, Massachusetts General Hospital. When I started my laboratory at MIT, I had little start-up money, and one student. I remember stating to the Dean at the time, that with so little in funding and support, it appeared he did not want me to succeed.

His response to me was "now you understand." This is perhaps to be discussed in my next book.

Nevertheless, beginning with a two-room lab and one student, working on an area that few thought would work (engineered bone regeneration), it is remarkable that fast forwarding I received 2021 the American Academy of Orthopaedic Surgeons Kappa Delta Award (highest research honor) for 30 years of research and achievement in bone regeneration research.

How did the NMA figure into this? Our very first work was trailblazing. We were able to isolate and grow bone cells on degradable polymers and show how and why the surfaces worked to support growth. We had just submitted the preliminary findings to the National Science Foundation for real funding of the work before we ran out our small amount of start-up funds from MIT. (We would eventually get the National Science Foundation funding that allowed our lab to continue based on the work, although NSF at the time expressed great incredulity that anyone could regenerate bone outside the body).

We decided to submit our work to a scientific meeting to present our findings. But where should we present? I remembered my mother and her great admiration for the National Medical Association. I looked up the organization and found they had a scientific assembly taking place in Las Vegas that year and that there was actually an orthopaedic surgery section to present papers which was my specialty choice.

At that point, I realized I had one huge problem: the lack of adequate financial support from MIT. Plane fare to Las Vegas, hotel and meals would be impossible to pay. Undaunted, I decided to contact the head of the orthopaedic surgery section of the National Medical Association. As was the custom, the section heads were often the leaders of the specialty area at one of the then two historically Black medical schools. Dr. Richard Grant was the Chair of Orthopaedic Surgery at Howard Medical School.

I called on a Friday afternoon. It began with "Hello this is Dr. Richard Grant," he said. "Dr. Grant, my name is Dr. Cato Laurencin, I'd like to present a paper at the NMA orthopaedic surgery section meeting in Las Vegas if I could," I replied. "Well, your timing is good, the deadline is next week and you can mail the abstract for me to review and I will decide if it will placed in the program" he stated. "Dr. Grant, I need to ask if there could be funding available for my presenting my paper. You see, I just completed my MD-PhD, I'm running my laboratory at MIT and also I'm a resident in Orthopaedic Surgery at Harvard and I don't think I have the funds otherwise to travel to Las Vegas." There was a pause. "Young man, I can tell you right now that the NMA has no funding to underwrite your presenting at our annual meeting," he said with great assurity. "However. you're running a lab at M.I.T. and you are in the Harvard Orthopaedic Surgery Program? Well, I on the other hand will pay all your expenses out of my own pocket just to see your face."

My first National Medical Association Meeting was an eye-opener. I presented my work in front of some of the greatest minds in orthopaedic surgery, all assembled at one place. I also was able to meet young physicians like me in the residency and fellowship phase of their training. In all, I counted my first experience with the National Medical Association as transformative for my life.

As for Dr. Richard Grant, I had a very short conversation with him at the end of the scientific meeting. He said he enjoyed meeting me, and I had done a wonderful job presenting my work. He then taciturnly asked, "How much were your costs?" I replied that airfare, hotel, and cabs for the week came to $950 dollars. He reached into his vest pocket and took out his checkbook. He completed a check for $950 and handed it to me. He then thanked me for coming to the meeting. I will never forget it.

My experience with the National Medical Association and Dr. Grant left three lasting impressions. First, I really enjoyed doing science, but I enjoyed sharing my work with others. The National Medical Association was a great venue to do so and I would continue to attend. Second, I was touched by the gesture of Dr. Grant in hosting me at the National Medical Association. I realized that my life had been blessed with people who knew little about me but had the faith and confidence to mentor me.

The episode at the NMA reinforced my desire to be a mentor and to give back to others. I would be especially approachable to anyone who would contact me out of the blue, as I did Dr. Grant. Third, an unexpected by-product of the National Medical Association meeting was interacting with people who were deeply passionate about the public health issues facing Black people. I had always had a bit of a passion for the area. In fact, while I majored in Chemical Engineering at Princeton, I also pursued a program in African-American Studies and received a certificate of proficiency in the area at graduation. So, I connected with people who connected with Black Racial Justice and Health issues.

I began to attend meetings of the National Medical Association each year, religiously. I would present at the orthopaedic surgery scientific section each year and, at the same time, drifted over to the House of Delegates to see the inner workings of the organization.

At the same, I drifted over to a new section of the organization, the resident (doctors in training) section. I happened to meet the leader of the section in the hall at the beginning of the NMA meeting. He was actually in his last year of residency and discussed the fact that the organization needed a resident-level person to work to lead the section. I counted the interaction as providence and immediately volunteered to take on the position.

I've learned in life that a number of opportunities come your way where swift decisions must be made. When the opportunities come, be bold, and you will almost never regret it. We walked around the corner into a large room filled with young people, like myself. The person accompanying me, the leader of the section, walked to the front of the room. I realized this was the resident section of the National Medical Association.

One of the first orders of business was an announcement by him of the next leader of the section. He stated in the absence of any new established procedures of election, the head of the section picks the next leader and that he had picked Dr. Cato T. Laurencin. I heard the crowd say "Who?" and from the back of the room, I raised my hand and waived. With that one step, I had been confirmed as the new leader of the resident section.

What I hadn't realized was that by leading the resident section, I became a member of the Board of Trustees for the entire National Medical Association. The Board had decided to create a temporary position a resident trustee until they fleshed out the language for a permanent person. So, at my second meeting at the National Medical Association, I became the leader of the residents, as well as a member of the board. My situation was a bit extreme, but not unusual. The NMA to this day is still an organization where young ambitious people can in a very short time take on important leadership roles in the organization.

Joining the board of the NMA in my 20s was of course "drinking from a fire hose" experience. Not only was I a fiduciary of the organization, but also I worked on important public health issues such as the future of Medicare, combatting HIV in the Black community and serving up information sources to members of the Congressional Black Caucus. What I really enjoyed about these early years of the National Medical Association was the mentorship. Senior Black physicians would treat me respectfully, but at the same time share their wisdom as a father or mother would do. I grew tremendously during my 4 years on the board of the National Medical Association.

I had grown up. I completed residency and had moved into fellowship and started my first job as a professor. But the NMA was still an important part of my life. My senior mentors at the NMA sat down with me after my last board member as the then legislated postgraduate trustee. They already had plans for me to be a delegate to the House of Delegates and had picked a committee and a council for me to take on senior leadership work at the national level. At the same time, I was advised to begin to work with my local society in Pennsylvania where I had taken a faculty position. "All politics are local," I was told, "And your future with the National Medical Association depends upon your work in your region."At the National Medical Association, there are no "chapters" per se. There are societies that are affiliated with the National Medical Association. They maintain their own charter and finances.

I returned to Philadelphia (to be discussed later) where I immediately joined the local society. My name was well known to all since my mother had been an active member of the society in her prime. The local society community was engaged.

Academics in the city of Philadelphia had an opportunity to present their work in a supportive venue. Those in private practice were able to obtain continuing medical education credits so vital for maintaining privileges at hospitals, for relicensure by the state, and increasingly for recertification by their specialty boards. All of us desired the friendliness and camaraderie found, whether it be to celebrate, commiserate, or something in between.

I was active in my local society and served on a variety of committees. I enjoyed the pleasure of doing good for my community from mentoring events to our annual scientific lecture day. I still, however, had a desire to work nationally with the National Medical Association. I remember at our national convention, some in my region questioned if I was ready to take on national responsibilities on the Board of Trustees. I was known as extremely active in my local areas but was thought to be unknown nationally. At the national convention, it became clear to all that I was a former trustee already (the postgraduate trustee). That knowledge and an understanding of the work I performed while a trustee cemented my election to Secretary of the House of Delegates (and membership to the Board of Trustees).

At the NMA, I worked my way from Secretary, to Vice-Speaker and then to Speaker of the House of Delegates of the National Medical Association. There, my passion for addressing health disparities and for promoting racial and ethnic diversity and justice was in full effect. Eventually I cofounded an institute on Black racial health disparities elimination, the W. Montague Cobb/NMA Health Institute, and became the editor in chief of its journal, the *Journal of Racial and Ethnic Health Disparities*.

My life and career in the area of promoting racial and ethnic health disparities elimination and the promotion of fairness and justice gained an exclamation point in my being awarded the Herbert W. Nickens Award from the American Association of Medical Colleges (AAMC). It was awarded for my work in promoting justice and fairness, work that began at the National Medical Association. I was honored to receive an award named after Dr. Herbert W. Nickens. He was someone ahead of his time, dedicated to issues of fighting racism and promoting inclusion. He passed at too young an age. While he was a "big" person in the field, he always took time to speak to young people like me when he was at the NMA. It left an important impression on me.

For my Herbert W. Nickens Award lecture, I had been thinking about what the future of both promoting diversity would be like and the future of addressing health disparities in the Black community would be like. In both cases, I felt that addressing racism in a learning environment that promoted antiracism would be the key in the future. I had previously written a paper entitled "Diversity 5.0" which stated that we needed to confront and address racism and discrimination if we wished create an American environment that had true diversity and inclusion. My address for the Herbert W. Nickens Award lecture laid out a blueprint for how we would achieve through what I called "The IDEAL Path." The talk was entitled, "Black Lives Matter in Science, Engineering and Medicine" and I share it with you here. "Good afternoon. I'm Dr. Cato Laurencin, and I am the University Professor and Albert and Wilda Van Dusen Distinguished Endowed Professor of Orthopaedic Surgery at the University of Connecticut. I am very proud to have received the Herbert W. Nickens Award of the American Association of Medical Colleges (the AAMC). I am equally proud to be able to provide this award lecture."

The title of my lecture is "Black Lives Matter Too in Science, Engineering, and Medicine."

"The death of George Floyd and so many, many others has provided new information and a new awakening on issues of racism in America. We've seen, in many ways, what amounts to a sea change in an understanding and appreciation of racism and its effects on America.[1]

When we use the term sea change, we are referring to a substantial change in perspective, which affects a society at large on a particular issue, and it can be considered to be similar to a paradigm shift. The term evolved from an older terminology meaning "change wrought by the sea."[1]

If we examine what's happening in terms of racism in America, one way is to examine Google searches. This slide shows the Google search activity for the term racism, either the word itself, or expanded versions, such as "what is racism."

Fig. 2.1 shows Google search activity for the term "racism," either the word itself or expanded versions such as "what is racism?"

What we see is that interest in concepts around racism tends to drop off every year in the summer, probably during vacation time, and the peaks are inconsistent, or less consistent, but they appear in November and April, and this is thought to be due partly to elections and primaries.[2]

What we do see is a sea change in levels of interest and concern about racism. This chart shows the tracking of racism searches before and after the passing of George Floyd since the start of 2020.

Fig. 2.2 shows the sea change after the passing of George Floyd, tracking racism searches since the start of 2020.

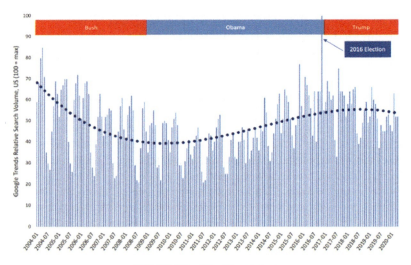

FIGURE 2.1 The ebb and flow

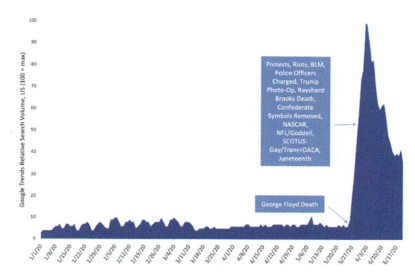

FIGURE 2.2   A sea change

What we can see is that there was a dramatic increase in searches after George Floyd died on May 25th of this year. Levels subsequently have moved to approximately 40% of the year's peak. Importantly, that 40% level is still over six times higher than the median interest in racism before May 25th.[2] So we are seeing a dramatic shift in concern and a desire for better understanding, in my opinion, regarding racism taking place in America.

The main thesis of my lecture today is that to truly combat health disparities in Blacks and to truly have Black diversity and equity exist, we must understand and combat racism. I'm going to provide a number of different articles that I've written over the years examining the intersection of health disparities, diversity, and racism. A paper I wrote called "Diversity 5.0: A Way Forward" describes the importance of combating racism if we are serious about moving forward with diversity.[3] The editorial entitled "The context of diversity," a piece I wrote in Science, which I'll refer to during my talk, discusses the need to again combat racism in terms of achieving diversity and the need for more precision in using the term diversity.[4]

"Racial Profiling Is a Public Health and Health Disparities Issue" was a paper that I recently wrote about racial profiling and its health effects on Black people and "A Pandemic on a Pandemic," a piece I wrote on racism and COVID-19 in Blacks in the journal *Cell Systems*, refers to the disparities taking place in COVID-19 and their root causes of racism.[5,6] Then in a new paper entitled Just in Time: Trauma Informed Medical Education, we discuss how bias and discrimination in our medical education establishments creates an unhealthy place to grow academically.[7] We adapt principles of the trauma-informed approach, first realizing this is occurring, recognizing the effects of bias and discrimination on students and trainees, responding with appropriate actions, and resisting retraumatization by creating a universal precaution environment and by addressing those who promulgate bias, discrimination, and racism.

In my lecture, I'd like to talk about racism and its history in America. I'd then like to talk about racism and its effects on the present day. I will discuss our modern definitions of racism and then how messages of racism continue to manifest themselves. My lecture will then discuss racial disparities and the correlates to racism. I will discuss allostatic load and racism. I'd then like to end by describing and discussing my new vision of the ideal pathway for us to pursue in terms of creating a just and diverse society.

Fig. 2.3 shows an outline of Dr. Cato T. Laurencin MD, PhD, to a just and diverse society, otherwise known as the inclusion, diversity, equity, antiracism, and learning (IDEAL) pathway.

Disparities in healthcare among Blacks have been known for a great deal of time. A landmark study done by the Institute of Medicine, now the National Academy of Medicine, produced very important study proceedings called "Unequal Treatment: Confronting Racial and Ethnic Health Disparities in Health Care." A key finding of the study was that racial discrimination was the major factor contributing to disparities in care in the setting of equal access.[8]

To quote from the Institute of Medicine report, "There is considerable empirical evidence that even well-intentioned whites who are not overtly biased and who do not believe they are prejudiced, typically demonstrate unconscious implicit negative racial attitudes and stereotypes."[8] A number of studies that they quoted in their study referred to this.

In one study examining Medicare beneficiaries enrolled in managed care plans, African-Americans were found to receive poorer quality of care in a variety of measures. This is very important because individuals in Medicare managed care plans will have equal access to care. This is a paper by Schneider that was published in *JAMA*.[9]

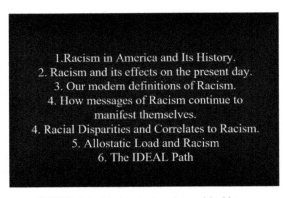

1. Racism in America and Its History.
2. Racism and its effects on the present day.
3. Our modern definitions of Racism.
4. How messages of Racism continue to manifest themselves.
4. Racial Disparities and Correlates to Racism.
5. Allostatic Load and Racism
6. The IDEAL Path

FIGURE 2.3 Racism in America and its history

Ryn and Burke found that doctors were more likely to ascribe negative racial stereotypes to their minority patients, despite controlling for differences in minority and nonminority patients' education, income, and personality characteristics.[10] Green et al. found the first evidence of unconscious implicit racial bias among physicians using a measure of implicit social recognition and described its predictive validity.[11]

The results of the Green study suggested that physicians' unconscious biases may contribute to racial and ethnic health disparities in the use of medical procedures such as thrombolysis in the treatment of myocardial infarction. The use of implicit bias testing has been done in a number of different settings after the study by Green, and by and large, has consistently found that these biases take place.[11] Unequal Treatment by the Institute of Medicine found that there is considerable empirical evidence that even well-intentioned whites who are not overtly biased and who do not believe they are prejudiced, typically demonstrate unconscious implicit negative racial attitudes and stereotypes.[8] Where else do we see the evidence of bias and racial discrimination against Blacks?

First, we can see where we've been as Black people in America. The cruelty of enslavement. I show a picture of a slave auction house here from the past.[12]

Fig. 2.4 shows "China, Glass, Auction & Negro Sales" in Atlanta, Georgia (1864) Photo by George N. Gardner.

The profound history of degradation of Black enslavement was followed by the rise and eventual fall of Jim Crow. Emancipation ended slavery, but not its legacy. Interestingly, Jim Crow was not a person, yet affected the lives of millions of people. This was named after a popular 19th-century minstrel song that stereotyped Black people. Jim Crow came to personify the system of government-sanctioned racial oppression and segregation in the United States. I refer you to the pbs.org website on Jim Crow on the rise and fall of Jim Crow as an era.[13]

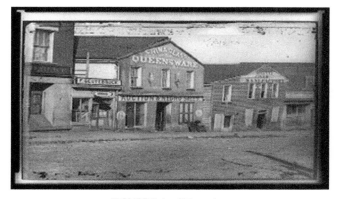

FIGURE 2.4 China, glass

Next came the Second Reconstruction that ended with the passage of the Voting Rights Act of 1965. During the period from the end of World War II until the late 1960s, referred to as the Second Reconstruction, the nation began to correct civil and human rights abuses that continued in American society for over a century.

These changes were really led by very courageous people in the civil rights movement. People like Rosa Parks who famously refused to give up her seat to a white passenger on a public bus in 1955. Her act of civil disobedience really galvanized the US civil rights movement in making the changes that were necessary.

So, the struggles of Black folks from slavery and legislated inequality have gone on from 1619 to 1965 and we must never forget. We must never forget the struggles that have taken place. This is a slide from a history book, a version of a history book that said the Atlantic slave trade between the 1500s and 1800s brought millions of workers from Africa to the southern United States to work on agricultural plantations.[14]

Fig. 2.5 shows an image from a history book that demonstrates the Atlantic slave trade between the 1500s and 1800s which brought millions of workers from Africa to the southern United States to work on agricultural plantations.

It's important that there isn't a revisionist history of slavery and the degradations that took place during time.

In the history of Black people in America, slavery and legislated inequality represent 85% of our history. There is much work that needs to be done to address, course correct, and move in right direction, as 85% of our history has been with slavery and legislated inequality.

Well, where are we now? Racism is a major driver of our culture. We can see it in the clothes and messaging placed on this young man. We can see it in messaging on food advertisements. This is a slide of a cereal box in which the only Black face or Brown face in the group is cleaning the floor.[15]

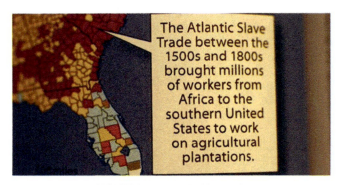

FIGURE 2.5   Atlantic Slave trade

Fig. 2.6A shows an image of a cereal box in which the only Black face or Brown face in the group is cleaning the floor, a clear racial message.

This was recently received by my wife. It was an advertisement from Barnes and Noble where one can choose The Bad Seed or The Good Egg as a book for children.[16] One can see the messaging that the bad seed is a black seed, and the good seed is a white egg. In America, we are bombarded with messaging regarding race in subtle and not so subtle ways.

Fig. 2.6B shows an advertisement received from Barnes and Noble which demonstrates the subtle and not so subtle race messaging conveying that the bad seed is a black seed, and the good seed is a white egg.

In discussing racism, I refer you to the great work of Dr. Camara Jones on levels of racism and her theoretical framework discussed in "A Gardener's Tale" where she eloquently defines the different types of racism and provides allegories as to how they are caused and what their manifestations are. Institutional racism is defined by her as differential access to the goods, services, and opportunities by race.

Institutional racism is often evident as inaction in the face of need. With institutionalized racism, there is an initial historical insult. There are structural barriers. There is as she said, inaction in the face of need. As a part of the result, there is unearned privilege that takes place.[17]

There is personally mediated racism with prejudice and discrimination.[17] Prejudice means differential assumptions about the abilities, motives, and intentions in others according to race. Discrimination means differential actions toward others according to race. This is commonly thought of in the term we know as racism.

As Dr. Jones discusses, personally mediated racism can be intentional or unintentional. It can involve acts of commission, or acts of omission. It maintains structural barriers and societal norms condone it.[17]

A.

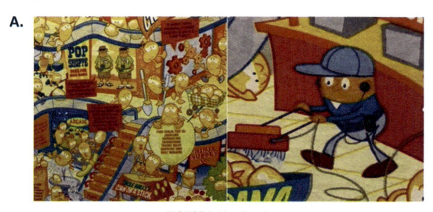

FIGURE 2.6A   Cereal

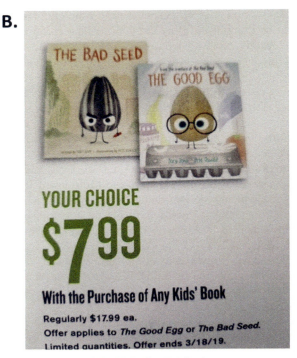

FIGURE 2.6B   Bad Seed

The third type of racism is internalized racism. It is defined as acceptance by members of the stigmatized race of negative messages about their own abilities and intrinsic worth. It's characterized by their not believing in others who look like them and not believing in themselves. Internalized racism reflects societal values.

It erodes the individual sense of value and undermines the collective actions of the group.[17]

Where else do we see evidence of bias and racial discrimination? Well, there are two examples that I think are important to note in our modern times. One is a struck down North Carolina voter ID law. This is a slide regarding the Supreme Court blocking a North Carolina voter ID law. A deadlocked Supreme Court refused to revive parts of a law, found to "target African-Americans with almost surgical precision."[18] The latest news is that this year an appeals court blocked yet another attempt to disenfranchise Black voters, and it is unlikely now that new restrictions will be in place in time for the upcoming election.

The Ally Bank case is a very well-known and famous case where a large settlement was made by Ally Bank to pay for a car loan bias. In the Ally bank case, individuals who were Black and Brown were charged higher interest rates than their scores indicated they should pay. The profit was split between

Ally Bank and also the dealers, clearly an example of racism and discrimination taking place.[19]

I sit on the Racial Profiling Prohibition Project Advisory Board for the State of Connecticut where we review data on disparities taking place in terms of traffic stops involving Black and Brown people. We know that, nationally in reviewing Justice Department statistics, a Black driver is 31% more likely to be pulled over than a white driver and 23% more likely than a Hispanic driver to be pulled over. In Connecticut, Black drivers are pulled over at higher rates for "pretext stops" (e.g., air freshener in rear view mirror, license plate abnormalities) than white drivers. The cars of Black drivers are searched at higher rates than white drivers, and those searches result in contraband at lower rates than white drivers.[20]

We've talked about the outside world. What about in terms of science, engineering, and medicine? I had the privilege of working on the Advisory Committee to the Director which had a working group on Diversity in the Biomedical Research Workforce. As discussed in the Chronicle of Higher Education, the NIH allocated $31 million to tackle the racial gaps in training.[21]

While there were a number of reasons why the racial gaps are taking place, there was also a disturbing discrepancy in success rates for research grants in applications from white and Black investigators. As reported by Ginther et al., this was found even after controlling for numerous observable variables.[22] While funding for increasing the number of investigators who can apply for grants is important and laudable, how discrimination and racism play a role in science and applications for federal funding must be studied further.

In clinical care, we know that there is a gap in terms of Black and white mortality. Between 1970 and 2004, it is estimated that 2.7 million excess Black deaths took place, making racism a more potent killer than prostate cancer, breast cancer, or colon cancer.[23] We know that combating racism can make a difference in the health of Blacks in America.

There's also the concept outside of the clinical setting, of just living as a Black person. Some people call it breathing while Black. This can be considered in the context of the allostatic load.

The allostatic load represents wear and tear on the body, which increases over time as an individual is exposed to repeated or chronic stress.[24] It represents a cycle of physiological consequences of chronic exposure to fluctuating or heightened neural and neuroendocrine responses that results from repeated or chronic stress. This term was coined by McEwen and Stellar in 1993.[25]

I serve as the editor in chief of the *Journal of Racial and Ethnic Health Disparities*. We published an important paper on racial discrimination and stigma consciousness associated with high blood pressure and hypertension in minority men. Stigma consciousness refers to individual differences in the extent to which targets believed that their stereotyped status pervades their interactions with members of other groups.[26]

In this study, lifetime racial discrimination and stigma consciousness were examined to ascertain associations with blood pressure in minority and white middle-aged and older white men. The conclusion was that discrimination and stigma consciousness were associated with common risk factors for chronic disease and premature death that disproportionately affect minorities.[26] Another study that was published in the *Journal of the National Medical Association* found that allostatic load burden can influence racial health disparities in levels of mortality. In this study, allostatic load burden partially explained higher mortality levels among Blacks independent of socioeconomic status and also health behaviors.[27]

So how does the allostatic load manifest itself as a Black person on a day-to-day basis? I am formally a professor at the University of Virginia and travel back to the area every couple of years. During my last visit, I saw an unprecedented number of bumper stickers all through my time driving through central Virginia portraying the Confederate flag. The Confederate flag for me hearkens back a time of enslavement, Jim Crow and continued racism. As a Black person, these may not only have personal emotional effects, but wear and tear health effects.

An article in the *American Journal of Hypertension* examined whether there was an association between race consciousness and the patient–physician relationship, medication adherence, and blood pressure in urban primary care of patients. In this study, that was done by Dr. Lisa Cooper; along with Dr. Camara Jones, race consciousness was defined as the constant psychological vigil and heightened physiological response associated with racial discrimination among Blacks. The hypothesis was that race consciousness could increase their risk of hypertension.

What they found was that, among Blacks, race consciousness was associated with a higher diastolic pressure.[28]

Where else have we seen dramatic health disparities take place? We've seen it in HIV/AIDS in the African-American community. I wrote a paper entitled "HIV/AIDS and the African-American Community 2018—a Decade Call to Action." As we know with recent statistics, Blacks represent, approximately, 13% of the US population, but in terms of diagnosed cases, 44% of the estimated new HIV diagnoses.[29]

An important study by clinicians at Johns Hopkins found that, at the height of the rise of HIV/AIDS, Blacks were treated differently than whites, in regard to antiviral prescribing. This was found in the setting of equal access and controlling for socioeconomic status. This raises the idea that the rapid increase in numbers of Blacks with HIV may be partly explained by differential treatment and racism that took place during that period of time.[30]

CDC projections right now are that 1 in 20 Black men will be HIV positive. 1 in 48 Black women will be HIV positive. 1 in 2 Black men who have sex with men will be HIV positive. 1 in 11 white gay and bisexual men will be HIV positive, and 1 in 99 Americans overall will be HIV positive.[31] HIV is at crisis levels in the Black community and so we must continue to address.

The Black male in America is particularly affected and at risk in a number of different ways. We've talked about HIV/AIDS, but let's discuss incarceration: America incarcerates people. Americans are 5% of the population, and 25% of the people incarcerated in the world.[32] Parenthetically, many of the countries with the lowest numbers of incarcerated individuals are actually on the continent of Africa. When we think about incarceration, right now 33% of those incarcerated in the United States are Black, way more than their proportion in the population.[33] Even beyond our discussion in terms of Black male incarceration, there are extensive data showing a punishing reach of racism for Black boys. New data show that 21% of Black men that were raised at the bottom of the socioeconomic order were incarcerated according to a snapshot of a single day during the 2010 census.[34]

An important study noted that the sons of Black families from the top 1% had about the same chance of being incarcerated on a given day as the sons of white families earning $36,000. As noted by Ibram Kendi, one of the most popular liberal, postracial ideas is that the fundamental problem is class, and not race.[34] Clearly this study explodes that idea.

I became very concerned about the fate of Black men in medicine. A number of studies and a number of our articles discussed the sharp drop in Black males in medical schools. In fact, one article said Black male doctors are becoming endangered.[35] They were, and they are.

We wrote a paper called, "An American Crisis—the Lack of Black Men in Medicine," and then proceeded working with the National Academies on an initiative to be able to create a workshop on Black men in medicine.[36] We, along with the W. Montague Cobb/NMA Health Institute, moved forward with a National Academy of Sciences, Engineering, and Medicine workshop on The Growing Absence of Black Men in Medicine and Science—An American Crisis. The workshop proceedings are available online for free at the National Academies Press.[37] I had the honor of chairing the workshop and was Rapporteur for the proceedings.

In the workshop proceedings, Dr. Victor Dzau, the President of the National Academy of Medicine, stated "This alarming trend threatens the quality of our health system, hampers progress in improving health for all, and challenges equity and justice." Dr. Camara Jones wrote, "Racism, this cultural morass of our nation, is a prime challenge and barrier for Black men along the trajectory."[37]

In discussing racism, one of the key effects that takes place is a disregard, disrespect, and dismissal of Black people in America. Perhaps this is why the Black Lives Matter movement has actually taken shape and grown because this is precisely what that movement is trying to address. The movement's purpose resonates with people, Black and white. So, as for racism, by naming it, learning about its past and present, and working to directly combat it, we may best address racial-based health disparities and also promote racial diversity.

Parenthetically, after our workshop that we had at the National Academy on Black men in medicine, we decided to move forward with a National Academies Roundtable on Black Men and Black Women in Science, Engineering, and Medicine. In my piece published in Science earlier this year, I wrote about the context of diversity and why we need initiatives such as this.[4]

In the piece entitled "The Context of Diversity," I referred to the fact that there are many groups that are under the diversity umbrella. With so many groups, it becomes easier for diversity efforts to disregard the historical and present drivers of discrimination and racism that the concept of diversity began with. In my piece, I wrote, "In other words, the greater context of inclusion and equity can get lost, making strides to diversify meaningless."[4]

I further wrote "This latter point is particularly relevant to Blacks in the United States who've experienced slavery, legally enforced segregation and discrimination, and now battle conscious and unconscious racism and mass incarceration. Institutionalized racism, past and present, has resulted in a disregard, disrespect, and dismissal of Black people from all walks of life. This is true in science, engineering, and medicine."[4]

So we've launched the Roundtable on Black Men and Black Women in Science, Engineering, and Medicine. I want to take this opportunity to thank the members of the steering committee who are on this slide, who first worked with me formulating this new entity.

These are the members of the roundtable.

Fig. 2.7A−C display the current members of the Roundtable for Black Men and Black Women in Science Engineering and Medicine.

There are 31 members, distinguished individuals, from across the country working in medicine, engineering, and science and who are like-minded in terms of the desire to move the needle forward quickly in addressing issues such as combating racism, improving health, and promoting diversity.

At the heart of the roundtable are what we call action groups. The aim of these action groups is to foster information sharing and the development of evidence-based approaches, along with engagement with key stakeholders in the broader community of scientists, clinicians, engineers, and administrators. The group works to design and conduct workshops, write papers, and conduct activities for meaningful change.

We have seven action groups right now. The first to be formed was the conscious and unconscious bias action group, addressing how to operate and identify mechanisms for intervention. Second, a pre-K to grad education action group was formed, which identifies disparities in education and the educational pipeline.

Third, there is a financing action group, which addresses the financial barriers to higher education and its impact. Fourth, there is a public advocacy, now called a public engagement action group, which determines how advocacy and public engagement can be utilized to bring issues of the roundtable to the forefront and to develop strategies for an increase in public awareness.

The National Academies of
SCIENCES · ENGINEERING · MEDICINE

Roundtable on Black Men and Black Women in Science, Engineering, and Medicine

Cato Laurencin, MD, PhD (NAE/NAM) *(chair)**
University Professor
University of Connecticut
Albert and Wilda Van Dusen Distinguished Professor
  of Orthopaedic Surgery
Professor of Chemical, Materials and Biomolecular
  Engineering
Director
Raymond and Beverly Sackler Center for
  Biomedical, Biological, Physical and Engineering
  Sciences
Chief Executive Officer
The Connecticut Convergence Institute for
  Translation in Regenerative Engineering

Olujimi Ajijola, MD, PhD
Assistant Professor of Medicine
UCLA Cardiac Arrhythmia Center
David Geffren School of Medicine at UCLA

Mark Alexander, PhD
Secretary
National Executive Committee, Health and Wellness
100 Black Men of America

Gilda Barabino, PhD (NAE)
Dean & Daniel and Frances Berg Professor
Office of the Dean
The City College of the CUNY

**Cedric Bright, MD, FACP *
Associate Dean for Admissions
Brody School of Medicine
East Carolina University

L.D. Britt, MD, MPH, D.Sc (Hon), FACS (NAM)
Henry Ford Professor and Edward J. Brickhouse
Chairman
Department of Surgery
Eastern Virginia Medical School

Kimberly Bryant
Founder and Executive Director
Black Girls CODE

Theodore Corbin, MD, MPP
Associate Professor of Emergency Medicine
Drexel University

Andre Churchwell, MD
Chief Diversity Officer
Vanderbilt University Medical Center
Senior Associate Dean for Diversity Affairs
Vanderbilt University School of Medicine
Professor of Medicine (Cardiology)
Professor of Radiology and Radiological Sciences
Professor of Biomedical Engineering

George Q. Daley, MD, PhD (NAM)
Dean of Faculty and Professor
Harvard Medical School

Wayne Frederick, MD, MBA
President
Howard University

Garth Graham, MD, MPH
President
Aetna Foundation

Paula T. Hammond, PhD (NAM/NAE)
David H. Koch Professor of Engineering
Department Head
Department of Chemical Engineering
MIT

Evelynn Hammonds, PhD, MS (NAM)
Barbara Gutmann Rosenkrantz Professor of
The History of Science
Professor of African and African American Studies
Chair, Dept of the History of Science
Harvard University

* denotes Steering Committee member

FIGURE 2.7A National Academies of Science

Fifth, the mentoring and advising action group examines and presents ideas on mentorship programs and pathways. Sixth, an action group on psychological factors examines the environment and stressors that take place with Black people in science, engineering, and medicine. Finally, a COVID-19 action group, examining COVID-19 in the Black community, has been formed.

The roundtable is responsible for conducting workshops, writing papers, and creating meaningful activities, and the action groups serve as the backbone of the roundtable in its functions throughout the year. The group convened our first meeting in December 2019, and we decided the first activity would be to discuss and address issues of racism.

The National Academies of
SCIENCES · ENGINEERING · MEDICINE

Ian Henry, PhD
Section Head, R&D Analytical Chemist
Proctor and Gamble

Camara Phyllis Jones, MD, MPH, PhD
Senior Fellow
Satcher Health Leadership Institute and
Cardiovascular Research Institute
Adjunct Associate Professor
Dept of Community Health and Preventive Medicine
Morehouse School of Medicine
Adjunct Professor
Dept of Epidemiology
Dept of Behavioral Sciences and Health Education
Rollins School of Publi c Health
Emory University

Orlando Kirton, MD, FACS, MCCM, FCCP, MBA
Surgeon-in-Chief, Chairman of Surgery
Chief Division of General Surgery
Abington-Jefferson Health
Vice Chairman
Jefferson Health Enterprise Dept of Surgery
Professor of Surgery
Sidney Kimmel Medical College
Thomas Jefferson University

John Lumpkin, MD, MPH (NAM)
Senior Vice President
Robert Wood Johnson Foundation

Shirley Malcom, PhD, MA (NAS)
Directorate for Education and HR Programs
AAAS

Cora Bagley Marrett, MA, PhD
Emeritus Professor
Department of Social Sciences
University of Wisconsin-Madison

Alfred M. Mays, MS
Program Officer
Burroughs Welcome Fund

Valerie Montgomery Rice, MD (NAM)
President and Dean
Office of the President and Dean
Morehouse School of Medicine

Randall C. Morgan, MD, MBA *
Executive Director
W. Montague Cobb/NMA Health Institute

Elizabeth Ofili, MD, MPH, FACC (NAM)*
Senior Associate Dean, Clinical Research Director
Clinical Research Center
Morehouse School of Medicine

Vivian W. Pinn, MD (NAM)*
Senior Scientist Emerita
Fogarty International Center
Former Director *(Retired)*
Office of Research on Women's Health
National Institutes of Health

Joan Y. Reede, MD, MS, MPH (NAM)
Dean for Diversity and Community Partenership
Associate Professor of Medicine
Dept of Medicine
Harvard Medical School

Louis Sullivan, MD (NAM)*
President Emeritus
Morehouse School of Medicine

Lamont R. Terrell, PhD
Head, R & D Talent and University Diversity
GlaxoSmithKline

Hannah Valentine, MD, PhD
Chief Officer for Scientific Workforce Diversity
NIH

* denotes Steering Committee member

FIGURE 2.7B   National Academies of Science

So, our first action group workshop was on racism. On April 13th and 14th, the workshop on The Impacts of Racism and Bias on Black People Pursuing Careers in Science, Engineering, and Medicine took place. The workshop examined the role of racism and bias in the decline of Black students in science, engineering, and medicine. It explored the historical trends of enrollment of Black students in medical, engineering, and science-based schools and also looked at ways to be able to address these issues.

This is the cover for the proceedings of the workshop.

The National Academies of
SCIENCES · ENGINEERING · MEDICINE

**Clyde W. Yancy, MD, MSc, MACC, FAHA, MACP,
FHFSA (NAM)**
Vice Dean, Diversity and Inclusion
Magerstadt Professor of Medicine
Professor of Medical Social Sciences
Chief, Division of Cardiology
Feinberg School of Medicine
Northwestern University
Associate Director
Bluhm Cardiovascular Institute
Northwestern Memorial Hospital
Deputy Editor
JAMA Cardiology

* denotes Steering Committee member

FIGURE 2.7C   National Academies of Science

Fig. 2.8 shows the cover of the proceedings of the workshop on The Impacts of Racism and Bias on Black People Pursuing Careers in Science, Engineering, and Medicine hosted by the Roundtable for Black Men and Black Women in Science, Engineering, and Medicine.

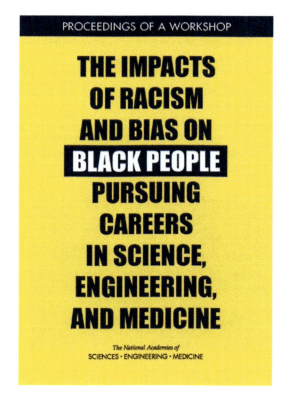

FIGURE 2.8   Impacts

The proceedings of the workshop on The Impacts of Racism and Bias on Black People Pursuing Careers in Science, Engineering, and Medicine will soon be available on the National Academies Press website as an e-book for free.[37]

Where should we be headed now? As I hope I am making clear, our understanding and appreciation of the impact of racism in America is vitally important. From there, anti-Black racism taking place in America must be understood. Anti-Black racism is the specific kind of racial prejudice directed toward Black people.

There's a very important piece entitled "A Reflection on Anti-Black Racism" by Marlysa Gamblin, which I'll be quoting and I refer you to the website in which it appears. "Anti-Blackness," she writes, "devalues Blackness while systematically marginalizing Black people, the issues that affect us, and the institutions created to support us. The first form of anti-Blackness is overt racism, which is upheld by covert structural and systemic racism that categorically predetermined the socioeconomic status of Blacks in this country. The second form of anti-Blackness is unethical disregard for Black people, as seen in the cases of police or civilian brutality against Black bodies."[38]

So what is the ideal path? I want to close by providing some of my vision for where I think we should move as a country in terms of issues of diversity and equity. Right now, discussions of diversity, inclusion, and equity are ubiquitous. While we have had some gains in these areas, they have not sufficiently addressed the issues of racism that we see in this country.

My belief is that we need to move to inclusion, diversity, equity, antiracism, and learning.

Fig. 2.9 shows IDEAL pathway to a just and diverse society, by Dr. Cato T. Laurencin, MD, PhD.

Antiracism according to Wikipedia is "a form of action against racism, systemic racism and the oppression of marginalized groups. Being antiracist is based on the conscious efforts and actions to provide equitable opportunities

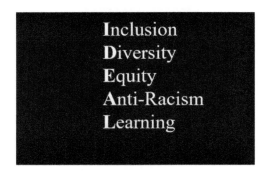

FIGURE 2.9   IDEAL

for all people on an individual and systemic level. People can act against racism by acknowledging personal privileges, confronting acts of racial discrimination and working to change personal racial biases."[39]

By learning, what do I mean? Understanding ways in which Black people are affected by the specific kinds of racial discrimination called anti-Blackness. Understanding the history of Black, Indigenous, and people of color. Moving from just an ally to what I would call a ride or die partner in the antiracism movement, these are some of the ways that I believe learning can be used in a constructive way to bring about the ideal pathway to move forward.

I'm very proud of our university, the University of Connecticut. We have just initiated a US Anti-Black Racism course. That course, which is now taking place and being offered to all faculty, staff, and students, is a one-credit course on the foundational history and concepts related to systemic and anti-Black racism.[40]

It's focused on the foundational concepts related to Black consciousness, Black resistance, Black resilience, and intersectional solidarity. It's particularly focused on the US context. It provides resources at UConn to continue the study, development, understanding, and potentially disrupting anti-Black racism for the collective good. Information on the course is available on the website of the Provost's Office at the University of Connecticut.[40]

This is the type of learning environment that can promote diversity, equity, and inclusion for all. Addressing antiracism is key in terms of moving forward as a nation and creating a more equitable environment. So, let's move from diversity, inclusion, and equity (DIE) to IDEAL.

Fig. 2.10 shows method of shifting from DIE to IDEAL pathway to a just and diverse society, by Dr. Cato T. Laurencin, MD, PhD.

I believe that's the pathway to the future.

I want to again give thanks to all for bestowing upon me the Herbert W. Nickens Award.[41] In this lecture, I have outlined my hope and vision for combatting racial and ethnic health disparities. I hope to be able to work with

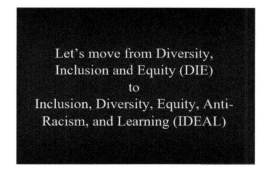

FIGURE 2.10 Let's Move From...

individuals across the country in the area of IDEAL, as we put into place an ideal path for achieving a better society.

Thank you.

My work in the area of pursuing racial justice and equity has taken me in a number of directions. In early March of 2020, I began seeing articles appearing on the Internet that suggested that Blacks could not contract the coronavirus. The origin of these articles was unknown to me. The sources were hard to track. Some stated that our melanin was protective of the coronavirus. Others stated that in China a Cameroonian was infected with the coronavirus early on and recovered rapidly from the virus. Others made an assumption that Blacks might have some resistance. For whatever the reason, I became worried that Black people might suffer from the virus at even higher rates. Blacks are disproportionately affected by poverty, mass incarceration, infant mortality, limited healthcare access, and health-related conditions including heart disease, diabetes, stroke, kidney disease, respiratory illness, and human immunodeficiency virus (HIV). Why then would we think that COVID-19 would affect us to a lesser extent than whites. Besides we knew that Blacks are more likely to work in service industry jobs that put workers in close contact with others. Blacks are overrepresented compared with the overall population in the food service industry, hotel industry, and taxi drivers and chauffeurs. This would make any social distancing more difficult. At the same time, we were beginning to see inconsistent information from government. Most Black Americans (60%) live in the south where guidance by governors on how to stay safe was inconsistent with the guidelines of the federal government. At the same time, my team and I saw a lack of reported and accessible data on the racial and ethnic composition of those infected. We understood that this might result in historically marginalized groups shouldering an even greater burden of disease and disproportionately bearing the social impact of disease.

After going to the state of Connecticut, Department of Health was able to obtain the first data on COVID-19 and its effects on the Black and Latino communities (Fig. 2.11).

The landmark paper was entitled the COVID-19 Pandemic: A Call to Action to Identify and Address Racial and Ethnic Disparities.

In our study, we reported that Blacks were contracting coronavirus infection and dying at higher rates than whites. This exploded the myth of Black immunity to the coronavirus. Subsequently, it was found that by the Centers for Disease Control and Prevention that while Black Americans comprised 33% of the hospitalizations in the COVID-19 Associated Hospitalization Surveillance Network (COVID-NET), they made up 18% of the analyzed population. In one study, majority Black counties had three times the rate of infections and six six times the rate of deaths as majority white counties.

My work has led me to demand that more be done to accurately collect and disseminate information on Black, Indigenous, and People of Color and

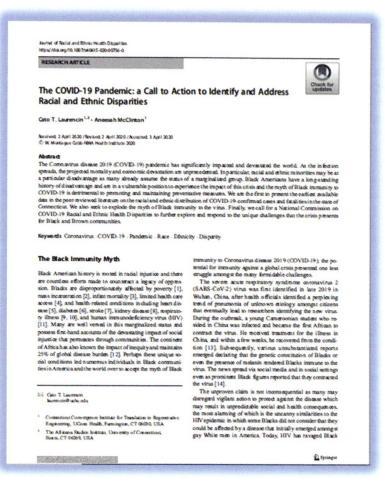

FIGURE 2.11 COVID

COVID-19. For that work, I was honored to be named a "Connecticut Healthcare Hero" by Connecticut Magazine. The article is featured as follows:

""Why in the case of an infection that we know disproportionately affects black people are we not adequately collecting data on black people?"

Back in February, if "Black" and "coronavirus" were typed into a search engine, some results would indicate Black people were resistant to COVID-19. A myth of Black immunity was circulating on the Internet and social media. Dr. Cato Laurencin, University Professor at UConn and CEO of the Connecticut Convergence Institute for Translation and Regenerative Engineering, was alarmed by what he found. "I set out to examine that because I was really concerned if that misinformation got out it could be disastrous for the black community," Laurencin says.

He requested data from the state on the number of infections and deaths by race and ethnicity, but was told they didn't have it. Laurencin pushed back, and in late March, he received the information. In late April, at the time of this interview, Laurencin said the state was still not consistently collecting race and ethnicity data. "It's unbelievable that we don't," Laurencin says. "That's a real issue that needs to be addressed today at a state and national level with the types of vigor that we do when we collect data on individuals who are incarcerated; we collect data by race and ethnicity on almost everything. But why in the case of an infection that we know disproportionately affects black people are we not adequately collecting data on black people?"

Laurencin knows COVID-19 disproportionately affects blacks because he and colleague Dr. Aneesah McClinton published the first peer-reviewed study in the nation with these findings in April. It exploded the myth and created an early warning that the disease could be particularly bad for the black community. In many ways, Laurencin says, Connecticut is a microcosm of America, especially in terms of the percentage of blacks in the overall population. (Blacks make up about 12% of Connecticut's population, according to US census data).

There were 96 deaths from COVID-19 in Connecticut at the time the study was published, and the trends were the same when that number hit 1000— Blacks were overrepresented in both cases and deaths. "Early on you collect the data, but No. 2, you also monitor and look at what the trends are," Laurencin says. "In this case the trends bear this out. There's also corroborating information from across the country with other centers such as Illinois and Wisconsin, which have also borne this out."

Laurencin says he believes that if data are properly presented, people will come around to understanding what's going on. Now there's a cacophony of voices saying there's a problem in the black community with COVID-19. "It's important to understand that the reason why the levels that we're seeing are this high is because of the history of discrimination that has taken place in this country," Laurencin says. "People say, 'Well, no, it's socio-economic.' Well, actually the socioeconomic portions of it are based upon the history of racism and discrimination in the country."

"People say, 'Well, it's the types of jobs people are doing.' Well, yes, but the types of jobs that people are doing are based upon the history of discrimination in the country. 'Well, maybe it's the housing situation people are in.' True, yes, it is partly the housing situation, but we have a history of housing discrimination and redlining that's taken place for a large number of years. And all of these come together as a perfect bad storm for Black people."

No matter how good you are at your job, or how many accolades and honors bestowed on you, it is important to ground that in your roots that gave you wings. They say that it is hard to be "it" if you've never seen it. I was fortunate to be raised by two amazing parents. I saw what it was like to be a doctor right with in the walls of our home. My mother was a brilliant physician who practiced on the first floor of our house in Philadelphia. There is one I know who has the combined grit, determination, and intelligence in quite the way that she did.

Her office had four parts: a waiting area, and office area for seeing patients, a procedure area for EKGs, etc., and a small laboratory for research. It was right there in our home that the spark of that being both a clinician and a scientist was born for me.

My father was a carpenter, a union man. He grew up in the island country of St. Lucia. He spoke French, was well learned, and yes, elegant in his speech and manner. Both my mother and my father taught me the same thing. "Always use your mind and your hands, and you will always have a good job." For my mother, it was about the laying on of hands as a physician. For my father, as a carpenter, the hands part was obvious. It was also about thinking and planning a construction project, and working out the goals and the timelines to make it happen.

Inspired by their lessons, I became an orthopaedic surgeon. Some say it was to please both my parents. But I really became an orthopaedic surgeon, because it was fun for me. I always say that an important goal in life is to do that you love so much that you would do it for free—but don't do it for free. Even though I knew that one day I would be a physician, I was drawn to chemical engineering during my undergraduate work at Princeton.

And when I started medical school at Harvard, one of my first goals to zero in on what was going to be my life's work as a physician. One option was to pick something in what we call the "ROAD": Radiology, Ophthalmology, Anesthesiology and Dermatology. These are great specialties, but what distinguishes them is that they have the ultimate ease of lifestyles. None were appealing to me.

To make a long story short, I simply loved orthopaedic surgery, where one takes care of people at all ages of the spectrum—young and old, and looks after their musculoskeletal needs. On the surface, orthopaedic surgery is simple. If something is broken, fix it. If something needs healing, your job is to help allow it to heal. A number of events cemented my desire to enter orthopaedic surgery. First, I met Dr. Henry Mankin, the Chair of Orthopaedic Surgeon at the Massachusetts General Hospital. He was full of personality and had a passion for both medicine and science, I immediately took to him. He took to me too, offering me a place to work in his laboratory separate from my work on my PhD at MIT at the time. He not only took me under his wing, but he still serves as a mentor and protector of sorts. I am forever grateful to him.

I think the most important thing he showed me is that one can be an orthopaedic surgeon and a scientist. At the time in which I was entering the field, the words orthopaedic surgeon and scientist were thought to be an oxymoron. He showed me that the terms were compatible.

After completing the Harvard Medical School (graduating Magna Cum Laude), I stayed on at Harvard for my orthopaedic surgery residency and eventually became Chief Resident in orthopaedic surgery at the Beth Israel Hospital/Harvard Medical School in Boston. The chiefship at Harvard was a tremendous experience. It was performed after residency was formally completed. Chiefs were what call "board eligible" and practiced and performed surgery completely on their own.

Fast forward, in addition to my work as a researcher and scientist, I am still an academic orthopaedic surgeon. I take care of patients, I still operate, and I teach orthopaedic surgery residents (doctors in training) and also teach medical students. My life as an academic orthopaedic surgeon is rewarding, and my career has included stints in private practice, as a Vice Chairman of the department, and also a Chairman leading faculty, staff, resident, and student. Combined with the other facets of my life, it is really rewarding.

I am a sport medicine and shoulder doctor. When I completed residency at Harvard, I spent a year as a fellow at hospital in New York called the Hospital for Special Surgery. It is an all-orthopaedic surgery hospital and it has probably the largest/finest collection of musculoskeletal surgeons that I have interacted with. The experience was transformative in terms of clinical skills and my ability to take on complex musculoskeletal cases.

I also had the great fortune of taking on being involved with lots of sports teams. In New York City, I was the assistant team doctor for the New York Mets, and went to Spring Training with them in Port St. Lucie, Florida. I moved to Philadelphia after my sports and shoulder fellowship and had a dream combination sports assignment. I was the doctor for my high school football team (Central High School) and took care of athletes in the large Community College of Philadelphia System in Philadelphia. But perhaps, my work in boxing has been the most interesting.

My work in boxing began in New York during my days as a fellow at the Hospital for Special Surgery. I met Dr. Barry Jordan, a fabulous neurologist who was a leader in the New York State Boxing Commission. I always loved boxing. I remember seeing bouts at Cloverlay gym in Philadelphia. I was particularly impressed by the tenets behind boxing: no drugs, no drinking, and no smoking, respect the body, and your grades count in school. Beyond all, the sportsmanship in boxing is unparalleled. It is not uncommon after a boxing match to see an opponent go to the opposite corner to thank his opponent's coach for training his opponent. The lessons for life are phenomenal.

I credit Dr. Jordan for getting me into boxing. While I was preparing to join the New York Boxing Commission, I moved to Pennsylvania. Barry Jordan was responsible for introducing me to the Pennsylvania commission. This led to my work as a ringside doctor not only in Pennsylvania, but also in New Jersey. With these credentials I was able to join USA Boxing. I've served as a doctor for USA Boxing for over 30 years and have served on their medical advisory board. I've been able to be the physician for the US Elite Men's Boxing Team, accompanying them to places around the world. It has been truly a rewarding experience. I believe it is part of my duty and service to my nation.

But a big part of my life has been in science and engineering. I'm not sure when I decided to devote a major part of my life to science. It started with my mother, and experiments taking place in her small laboratory at my house. It was cemented by meeting Dr. Robert Langer, my mentor who showed me where science could take the world. Along the way, there have been countless others, some that I will mention later, including Dr. Judah Folkman that have shaped me and my career.

As a professor in engineering and science, I conduct groundbreaking research, I run a large research center, and I teach. Each part of the job is exhilarating. For instance, in teaching, I was fortunate to obtain funding from the National Science Foundation. We bring Hartford City high school students and Hartford high school teachers to work in our laboratories each summer. The teachers are superbright. They have even published articles based on their work for just a summer. At the same time, we have undergraduate students, graduate students pursuing master's degrees, graduate students pursuing PhDs, and postdoctoral fellows who have already completed degrees while working under me.

I started working in a field known as tissue engineering in 1987 when I finished my PhD. It was a new field. In fact, Professor YC Fung is credited with naming the field in 1986/1987, stating, "we should name this new area that we are doing, tissue engineering." I define tissue engineering "the application of biological, chemical, and engineering principles toward the repair, restoration, or regeneration of living tissues using biomaterials, cells, and factors alone or in combination." I created this definition about 20 years ago, and it is still consistent to this day.

While the area of tissue engineering has had its advances, I as stated in the first part of the book, I think we can do much more. So, I thought long and hard about how we can rapidly progress the field. At the same time, I and others began to discuss that some of the great progress in science will come at the interface of medicine, biology, physics, and engineering. The convergence of these areas, if you will, will produce new advances in technology and science. I was fortunate to contribute to the national dialogue on convergence through a national academies workshop on the area. We defined convergence as simply the "The coming together of Insights and Approaches from Originally Distinct Fields."

Eventually I decided to put together my vision for the future of engineering tissues through approaches that embrace convergence. I took a page from Dr. Fung. Just as he named a new field, I decided to name my own. I decided to name the new field, "Regenerative Engineering." And it stuck.

Next, as "Fortune Favors the Prepared Mind" as stated by Louis Pasteur, I was approached by the editors of *Science Translational Medicine*. They began to hear of my vision of a new field and were intrigued enough to ask me to discuss my vision, which I did in a piece in Science Translation.

Our modern definition of regenerative engineering is the convergence of advanced materials science, stem cell science, physics and developmental biology, and clinical translation toward the regeneration of complex tissues, organs, or organ systems (Figs. 2.12 and 2.13).

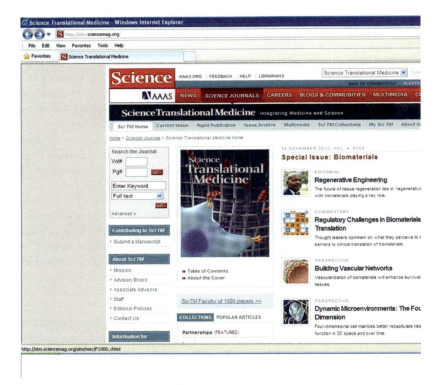

FIGURE 2.12   Scientific translation

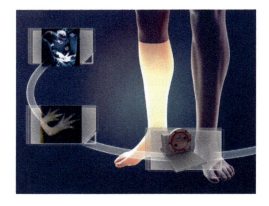

FIGURE 2.13   Regenerative engineering

The field combines together and creates totally new toolbox for tissue regeneration. It is one that we didn't have 30 years ago. It combines nanotechnology material systems which we did not appreciate until work from my group and other used nanotechnology-based material systems in the 1990s, and stem cell science which has really grown to be a mature field over the past 20 years. We have really grown to appreciate how physical forces govern regeneration. I believe it will be crucially important in solving grand challenges.

We have always appreciated developmental biology and morphogenesis and how animals regrow their lost limbs. But how do we bring it together with other technologies is a goal. And finally, most scientific fields have clinicians attached to the work as an afterthought. As an engineer—clinician—scientist, I think this a drawback in many fields. Clinicians must be full partners in the science being conducted.

We have come a long with our new field of regenerative engineering. As I stated, we define it as "The Convergence of advanced materials science, stem cell science, physics, developmental biology and clinical translation toward the regeneration of complex tissues, organs, or organ systems." We have a textbook of *Regenerative Engineering*, a journal *Regenerative Engineering and Translational Medicine*, and the Regenerative Engineering Society that is dedicated to promoting the field with engineers, clinicians, and scientists all working together. We believe in developing the next generation of a new type of engineer, ones that are skilled in convergence research.

And we have developed a master's in science degree program in regenerative engineering, and after applying to the National Institutes of Health, we received a large grant to train the next generation of scientists in our new field of regenerative engineering. Equally gratifying is the fact that we have other universities following suit and developing programs in regenerative engineering. At the same time that we received a training grant for regenerative engineering, Northwestern University had its training grant funded in regenerative engineering by a different institute inside of the National Institutes of Health. The new field aimed at addressing grand challenges such as limb regeneration truly has legs (please excuse the pun).

To summarize, to regenerate a limb, this is the opportunity that regenerative engineering offers us. The multiyear, multidimensional quest for this most ambitious goal has just been launched with the prospect of redefining the clinical treatment of musculoskeletal disease.

I want to share with you a great article written by my friend Melba Newsome that describes the prospects for my work.

"Regrowing Amputated Limbs Is Getting Closer to Medical Reality"— Melba Newsome Kirstie Ennis, an Afghanistan veteran who survived a helicopter crash but lost a limb, pictured in May 2021 at Two Rivers Park in Colorado.

"In June 2012, Kirstie Ennis was 6 months into her second deployment to Afghanistan and recently promoted to sergeant. The helicopter gunner and seven others were 3 hours into a routine mission of combat resupplies and troop transport when their CH-53D helicopter went down hard.

Miraculously, all eight people onboard survived, but Ennis' injuries were many and severe. She had a torn rotator cuff, torn labrum, crushed cervical discs, facial fractures, deep lacerations, and traumatic brain injury. Despite a severely fractured ankle, doctors managed to save her foot, for a while at least.

In November 2015, after 3 years of constant pain and too many surgeries to count, Ennis relented. She elected to undergo a lower leg amputation but only after she completed the 1000-mile, 72-day walking with the wounded journey across the United Kingdom.

On Veteran's Day of that year, on the other side of the country, orthopaedic surgeon Cato Laurencin announced a moonshot challenge he was setting out to achieve on behalf of wounded warriors like Ennis: the Hartford Engineering A Limb (HEAL) Project.

Laurencin, who is a University of Connecticut professor of chemical, materials, and biomedical engineering, teamed up with experts in tissue bioengineering and regenerative medicine from Harvard, Columbia, UC Irvine, and SASTRA University in India. Laurencin and his colleagues at the Connecticut Convergence Institute for Translation in Regenerative Engineering made a bold commitment to regenerate an entire limb within 15 years—by the year 2030.

"Regenerative Engineering—A Whole New Field"

Limb regeneration in humans has been a medical and scientific fascination for decades, with little to show for the effort. However, Laurencin believes that if we are to reach the next level of 21st-century medical advances, this puzzle must be solved.

An estimated 185,000 people undergo upper or lower limb amputation every year. Despite the significant advances in electromechanical prosthetics, these individuals still lack the ability to perform complex functions such as sensation for tactile input, normal gait and movement feedback. As far as Laurencin is concerned, the only clinical answer that makes sense is to regenerate a whole functional limb.

Laurencin feels other regeneration efforts were hampered by their siloed research methods with chemists, surgeons, and engineers all working separately. Success, he argues, requires a paradigm shift to a transdisciplinary approach that brings together cutting-edge technologies from disparate fields such as biology, material sciences, physical, chemical, and engineering sciences.

As the only surgeon ever inducted into the academies of science, medicine, and innovation, Laurencin is uniquely suited for the challenge. He is regarded as the founder of regenerative engineering, defined as the convergence of advanced materials sciences, stem cell sciences, physics, developmental biology, and clinical translation for the regeneration of complex tissues and organ systems.

But none of this is achievable without early clinician participation across scientific fields to develop new technologies and a deeper understanding of how to harness the body's innate regenerative capabilities. "When I perform a surgical procedure or something is torn or needs to be repaired, I count on the body being involved in regenerating tissue," he says. "So, understanding how the body works to regenerate itself and harnessing that ability is an important factor for the regeneration process."

The Birth of the Vision

Laurencin's passion for regeneration began when he was a sports medicine fellow at Cornell University Medical Center in the early 1990s. There he saw a significant number of injuries to the anterior cruciate ligament (ACL), the major ligament that stabilizes the knee. He believed he could develop a better way to address those injuries using biomaterials to regenerate the ligament. He sketched out a preliminary drawing on a napkin one night over dinner. He has spent the next 30 years regenerating tissues, including the patented L-C ligament.

As the chair of Orthopaedic Surgery at the University of Virginia during the peak of the wars in Iraq and Afghanistan, Laurencin treated military personnel who survived because of improved helmets, body armor, and battlefield medicine but were left with more devastating injuries, including traumatic brain injuries and limb loss.

"I was so honored to care for them and I so admired their steadfast courage that I became determined to do something big for them," says Laurencin.

When he tells people about his plans to regrow a limb, he gets a lot of eye rolls, which he finds amusing but not discouraging. Growing bone cells was relatively new when he was first focused on regenerating bone in 1987 at MIT; in 2007, he was well on his way to regenerating ligaments at UVA when many still doubted that ligaments could even be reconstructed. He and his team have already regenerated torn rotator cuff tendons and ACL ligaments using a nanotextured fabric seeded with stem cells.

Even as a finalist for the $4 million NIH Pioneer Award for high-risk/high-reward research, he faced a skeptical scientific audience in 2014. "They said, 'Well what do you plan to do?' I said, 'I plan to regenerate a whole limb in people.' There was a lot of incredulousness. They stared at me and asked a lot of questions. About 3 days later, I received probably the best score I've ever gotten on an NIH grant."

In the Thick of the Science

Humans are born with regenerative abilities—2-year-olds have regrown fingertips—but lose that ability with age. Salamanders are the only vertebrates that can regenerate lost body parts as adults; axolotl, the rare Mexican salamander, can grow extra limbs.

The axolotl is important as a model organism because it is a four-footed vertebrate with a similar body plan to humans. Mapping the axolotl genome in 2018 enhanced scientists' genetic understanding of their evolution, development, and regeneration. Being easy to breed in captivity allowed the HEAL team to closely study these amphibians and discover a new cell type they believe may shed light on how to mimic the process in humans.

"Whenever limb regeneration takes place in the salamander, there is a huge amount of something called heparin sulfate around that area," explains Laurencin. "We thought, 'What if this heparin sulfate is the key ingredient to allowing regeneration to take place?' We found these groups of cells that were interspersed in tissues during the time of regeneration that seemed to have connections to each other that expressed this heparin sulfate."

Called GRID (groups that are regenerative, interspersed, and dendritic), these cells were also recently discovered in mice. While GRID cells don't regenerate as well in mice as in salamanders, finding them in mammals was significant.

"If they're found in mice. we might be able to find these in humans in some form," Laurencin says. "We think maybe it will help us figure out regeneration or we can create cells that mimic what grid cells do and create an artificial grid cell."

What Comes Next?

Laurencin and his team have individually engineered and made every single tissue in the lower limb, including bone, cartilage, ligament, skin, nerve, and blood vessels.

Regenerating joints and joint tissue is the next big mile marker, which Laurencin sees as essential to regenerating a limb that functions and performs in the way he envisions.

"Using stem cells and amnion tissue, we can regenerate joints that are damaged, and have severe arthritis," he says. "We're making progress on all fronts, and making discoveries we believe are going to be helping people along the way."

That focus and advancement is vital to Ennis. After laboring over the decision to have her leg amputated below the knee, she contracted MRSA 2 weeks postsurgery. In less than a month, she went from a below-the-knee-amputee to a through-the-knee amputee to an above-the-knee amputee.

"A below-the-knee amputation is night-and-day from above-the-knee," she said. "You have to relearn everything. You're basically a toddler."

The clock is ticking on the timeline Laurencin set for himself. Nine years might seem like forever if you're doing time but it might appear fleeting when you're trying to create something that's never been done before. But Laurencin isn't worried. He's convinced time is on his side.

"Every week, I receive an email or a call from someone, maybe a mother whose child has lost a finger or I'm in communication with a disabled

American veteran who wants to know how the progress is going. That energizes me to continue to work hard to try to create these sorts of solutions because we're talking about people and their lives."

He devotes about 60 hours a week to the project and the roughly 100 students, faculty and staff who make up the HEAL team at the Convergence Institute seem acutely aware of what's at stake and appear equally dedicated.

"We're in the thick of the science in terms of making this happen," says Laurencin. "We've moved from making the impossible possible to making the possible a reality. That's what science is all about."

Will it be difficult to achieve, yes, but my philosophy has been that life is about triumphs, opportunities, challenges, and trials, and that success in life is about addressing each of these head on.

I embrace challenges. Bob Marley once said, "You never know how strong you are until strong is your only choice. Challenges build you, they make you better.

Always embrace challenges, they turn in to opportunities that turn in to triumphs.

This book is in large part about explaining my philosophy. It begins with simple words—Be bold, and take chances.

Now when I state, be bold and take chances, I do mean with some level of common sense. I don't advocate trying to traverse the Grand Canyon for instance (except if you are Evil Knievel and getting paid). But measured quality chances are necessary to be successful in life.

There are six major traits that I think are important to be successful. They are as follows:

Be smart.
Be hard working.
Be a good person.
Be loyal.
Be courageous.
Be adaptable and resilient.

Be Smart

Being smart serves as a buffer for the negativity that is bound to come your way in life. I was a professor at the University of Virginia for a number of years. I love the school and the academic environment. As an emeritus professor there, I often remember speeches that would start from a quote from Thomas Jefferson. Although parts of his history are troubling to me, there is no doubt there were aspects of him and his thought processes that were extraordinary. Jefferson stated in 1817, "Knowledge is Power, Knowledge if Safety. Knowledge is Happiness. As I have gotten older and a bit wiser, I have come to appreciate this quote. Being smart is not just about being intelligent, it is about cultivating those things about you that make you special as a smart individual. I had the honor of being a university professor at the University of Virginia, an elite group of academicians who reported to the President of the University of Virginia."

One of my colleagues was Professor Anita Jones who served in leadership positions in our nation's defense through science. She taught me (and others). "If you're going to compete, make sure you have an unfair advantage." What is an unfair advantage might you ask. An unfair advantage is an advantage that you have, that others don't have, and others never will. Homing in on what your unfair advantages are and then cultivating them is a key factor for success. I talk about this in more detail in the last section of this book.

And I can tell you that some people don't like the term "unfair" advantage because it sounds as if, well, it sounds as if it unfair. I once gave a speech in which Dr. Jones was present and used the phrase "if you're going to compete, make sure you have a super advantage." I was called out by Dr. Jones in the crowd when she stated "no, the term is 'unfair' advantage," and so I will not deviate from her instructions.

What is an example of an unfair advantage? I'm a chemical engineer, I'm a surgeon, and I'm a materials scientist. As an engineering, physician, and scientist, I exist in the world that few (humbly said) can match my background. That is an unfair advantage I use when formulating grants for funding, for writing papers, for planning my research, and in thinking about the care of my patients.

Identifying, cultivating, and utilizing your unfair advantages are a special key for success.

Be Hard Working

I've found that working hard has its benefits. I am constantly reminded by the poem of Langston Hughes titled Mother to Son.

"Well, son, I'll tell you: Life for me ain't been no crystal stair. It's had tacks in it, And splinters, And boards torn up, And places with no carpet on the floor"—Bare.

But all the time I'se been a-climbin' on, And reachin' landin's, And turnin' corners, And sometimes goin' in the dark. Where there ain't been no light.

So boy, don't you turn back. Don't you set down on the steps 'cause you finds it's kinder hard. Don't you fall now—For I'se still goin', honey, I'se still climbin', And life for me ain't been no crystal stair. Ain't been no crystalstair."

People I have admired the most, people I emulate, have been those who have worked hard, and that's probably why it comes natural to me. For me, life hasn't been a crystal stair. But for most people who are successful, it isn't for them either.

One of the things I teach though is to not confuse activity for accomplishment. All activities, efforts, and hard work should be purposeful. The legendary singer, James Taylor who I've met, and is a story for another book, once wrote in a song:

"It seems 'learn not to burn' means to turn on a dime and walk on if you're walking even if it's an uphill climb. And try to remember that working's no crime, just don't let 'em take and waste your time."

Luck is important in life. Being at the right place at the right time and gaining advantages from that can be significant. But it has been said, and it is true for me that "the harder I work, the luckier I get."

Working hard and addressing problems head on are important. Each morning I create a "To-Do" list of things to be accomplished each day. I like To-Do lists.

Often through whirlwind days, one can ask, "What have I accomplished?" To-Do lists help to answer that. I rank the things to do by their level of difficulty. It is too easy to create a list and work off of the low hanging fruit. The main reason is that it is too easy sometimes for big issues to slip through the cracks only to return later with a vengeance. I have found that problems that go away by themselves usually come back by themselves. The bigger the problem, the stronger the return. So, I rank what needs to be accomplished by the importance of the problem and not the ease of the solution.

Be a Good Person

Being a good person is important, no matter who you are or how important your job is. That may sound simplistic, but it is a simple truth. As a university professor, I remember my exit interview with John Casteen, the President of the University of Virginia. I greatly admire President Casteen. He has a big heart and he is hugely smart. I had just taken a Vice President position at the University of Connecticut, and I was having my exit discussion with him at his home. He gave me an important piece of information that was easy to absorb, because it embodied my philosophy, but it was good hearing it from him. He told me that there were three things that were key for life: (1) when you open your mouth, make sure everything you say is true; (2) it's important to know that you don't have to tell everyone, everything you know all the time; and (3) importantly, take time to go the bathroom. He said number 3 to me with a wry smile. I found all three lessons to be important.

It's important to be good person for the simple fact that every morning you walk to a mirror and see yourself. You have to like what you see. You have to like what you stand for. You have to like what you are becoming. Being a good person is something I look for in people. I try to surround myself with those individuals.

Be Loyal

As I have grown older and older, I value loyalty more and more. I have been fortunate to be blessed with people around me who are truly loyal. Professor Lakshmi Nair, Professor Yusuf Khan, and Professor Kevin Lo have been my students, and they stayed with me through multiple career moves and are not only loyal, good, and salt of the earth people, but they are exceptionally bright and hardworking scientists in their own rights. Loyalty is something that I look for in people. It can't be taught and can't be made up for if it is lacking. It is difficult for me to work with individuals who are not loyal.

Perhaps this is something that I should be able to do, but at this point in my career, I place such a high premium on loyalty that I stress that in all my relationships.

Be Courageous

Success is about courage. It is about making courageous decisions and courageous choices. It is about learning to take chances and learning to deal with the results: the positive and sometime not so positive choices. Maya Angelou once said, "I believe that the most important single thing, beyond discipline and creativity is daring to dare." I say, without courage, there is no progress.

But courage can be tough. Emerson stated, "Whatever course you decide upon, there is always someone to tell you that you are wrong. There are always difficulties arising which tempt you to believe that your critics are right. To map out a course of action and follow it to an end requires courage."

Lurking in the shadows, preventing courageous decisions is the fact that things may not work out, or to use the "F" word, you may **fail**. Let me provide a bit of philosophy that may help temper these feelings.

I've called it the Laurencin 15%−30% rule. It states that 15%−30% of the things you strive to achieve in life should **not** work out. Because it means THAT YOU ARE STRIVING. If everything you attempted to achieve, you succeeded at means YOU ARE NOT STRIVING ENOUGH. Why 15%−30%? Well, if it was a 60% rule, it might lead to depression, since that would mean that the majority of things you strive for would not work out. But the 15%−30% level is an important range that means you are going about life in the right way, a righteous way, and in a courageous way.

There are three major ways that things do not work out and my thoughts on them. The 15%−30% rule takes place in a type A decision world. This a world in which one makes a decision in striving for something good or great. You thought it was a good thing to do, and at the time, it was a good thing to do. As stated earlier, this a good thing because it means you are striving or stretching yourself. There are type B decisions that we make.

These are the decisions that you truly feel are the right thing to do. They turn out to not be the right thing to do, for any of various reasons, including having wrong information, or impulsiveness on your part, etc. While these might not be the best things, they are ok to encounter, because one can learn from the experiences and the experiences can help you the next time, especially if you reencounter the experience. Then there are type C decisions.

These are the decisions that you start off believing are wrong to make at this point in time. For some reason, you decide or are persuaded to follow a path that you know will not be successful or that you should not do. They turn out to not be the right thing to do for various reasons. These are decisions to avoid, since one gains nothing from a bad outcome from a decision one knew was wrong. But I think it is important to step out on the best knowledge you have at the time and decide.

Be Adaptable and Resilient

Adaptability allows for success to occur. Resiliency serves as an insurance policy for success. When I was growing up, I always heard of sayings of Charles Darwin. The quote he had was "Survival of the Fittest." But actually, what Darwin really said was "It's not the strongest of the species that survives, nor is it the most intelligent. It is the one that is most adaptable."

Adaptability allows one to be to assess situations and make new plans regarding them. To further elucidate this, I want to go back to my ringside boxing days. I've been fortunate to be a ringside boxing doctor at the professional level and at the amateur level. I've actually been a Commissioner of Boxing for the state of Connecticut because of my interest in the sport, especially in making it safer. I always marvel at the way in which professional boxers approach a fight they are constantly examining what they are doing and looking for ways to adapt to their opponents' tactics (Fig. 2.14).

The person who I think did that with great expertise over the years was Mike Tyson, with whom I had the opportunity to serve as a ringside boxing doctor for one of his championship fights.

Mike Tyson has developed a fabulous career in acting, beyond his life in the ring. His one-person play was extraordinary. He's also developed into a bit of philosopher. He got a plan for his next acts and rebuilding and it is working for him.

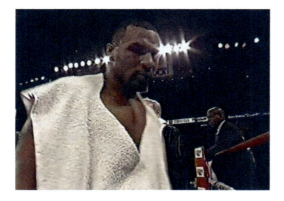

FIGURE 2.14 Mike Tyson

I am a strong advocate for creating a plan. It should be a long-term plan, a medium-term plan, and a short-term plan. The short-term plan should be the daily To-Do list, which I described to you. But it is important to remember the philosophy of Charles Darwin, which stresses the importance of adaptability. It is also important to remember Mike Tyson's philosophy when he says:

Everybody has a plan until they get punched in the face.

Mike Tyson.

The ability to adapt to new conditions (the punch in the face) is crucially important to success, in your career and in your life. Equally, if not more important, is building resiliency. In the boxing analogy, this is the ability to take a punch, be knocked down and get back up again. Resiliency just doesn't occur. It takes years of preparation, and also it takes exposure to incidences where you have to be down and get back up. Remember that life is about triumphs, opportunities, challenges, and trials, and they all must be embraced. My embracing all facets of life, I can tell you that my resiliency has been built over time, and experience. To paraphrase Drizzy Drake (one of my favorite artists): "I'm on a roll like Cottenelle, because I was made for all this [stuff]." It says a lot about the ability to look the tough stuff in the face and keep moving forward. It's powerful.

Those are my basics tenets, and they just scratch the service. But they will serve you well if you practice them with commitment and intention, but let's did a bit deeper.

Be Appreciative, Remember the Past, and Always Move Forward

This has been an important part of my philosophy of life. I had the great opportunity to express this in winning the Spingarn Medal. The Spingarn is the highest award given by the National Association for the Advancement of Colored People (NAACP). The Spingarn Medal is given for outstanding achievement by an African American. The award was created in 1914 by Joel Elias Spingarn, chairman of the board of directors of the NAACP. It was first awarded to biologist Ernest E. Just in 1915 (for whom I received another award named after him in 2019) and has been given most years thereafter. As the story goes, in 1913, Spingarn, a white man, traveled across the United States to recruit members to the NAACP. Reading local newspapers in many cities, he saw that the media focused on negative portrayals of African-Americans. He established the Spingarn Medal in 1914 to provide national attention to the impressive contributions of African-American citizens and to counter the media's racist stereotyping. The goal of the award is to increase the racial pride of African-Americans and to stimulate the ambition of African-American youth. The importance of the impact of the award is as relevant now as it was over 100 years ago. I am proud to be the 106th Spingarn medalist, given to me in July of 2021.

The Encyclopedia Britannica has the original award. It states that the Spingarn Medal is a gold medal awarded annually by the National Association for the Advancement of Colored People, since 1915 to honor "the man or woman of African descent and American citizenship who shall have made the highest achievement during the preceding year or years in any honorable field."

I share with you my acceptance remarks.

"I want to first begin by thanking the leadership of the NAACP, especially the Spingarn Award Committee, for selecting me to receive this singular honor which is the Spingarn Medal. I want to thank Dr. Dwayne Proctor, Chair of the NAACP Foundation, and Mr. Scott Esdaile, the President of the Connecticut NAACP, my brothers in arms, for their friendship and support.

I want to thank the great Professor Robert Langer, a chemical engineer, and my mentor. I want to thank and pay tribute to Dr. Louis Sullivan who introduced me. He is a tremendous physician—scientist and administrator who has helped pave the way for me and many others. Dr. Langer and Dr. Sullivan, I appreciate both of you.

The list of those who have won the Spingarn Medal is incredible and includes Dr. Martin Luther King, Jr., George Washington Carver, Ernest Just, Percy Julian, and the great Maya Angelou. I am honored to be in such awesome company.

I want to pay homage to those who have come before me. Maya Angelou wrote, "I am a Black Ocean, leaping and wide. Welling and swelling I bear in the tide.

Bringing the gifts that my ancestors gave. I am the dream and the hope of the slave. I rise.

I rise, I rise."

From Cato, who led the Cato Rebellion in South Carolina in 1741, to Cato Wilson, born in Georgia in 1811, to Cato Wilson, my namesake, a class of 1895 graduate of Meharry Medical College, thank you. Thank you for your persistence, your perseverance, and your determination.

I want to thank my father Cyril Laurencin, a strong union carpenter, and my mother Dr. Helen I. Moorehead Laurencin, a trailblazer in medicine and science and a leader of her community in North Philadelphia.

My parents taught me Black Excellence. My parents taught me Black Resilience. Because of them, to paraphrase Drizzy Drake, "I'm on a roll like Cottenelle, because I was made for all this stuff."

Moving now to the present, I pay homage to my wife Cynthia and my beautiful and intelligent children. Thank you, I love you, you motivate me each day to strive. And to my many colleagues and students, I share this day, and this award with you.

I had the honor of winning Africa's Science Prize, the UNESCO Equatorial Guinea International Prize for Research in the Life Sciences. I shared it with among others, Tu Youyou, the first woman from China to win the Nobel Prize.

I am the first person from the African diaspora to receive this award. When I addressed the leaders of the African Union last year in Ethiopia, I stated that we need to create new initiatives uniting Black people throughout the world in the pursuit of engineering, medicine, and science. A daunting task yes, but there is a Massai proverb that states, "The village which is not discussed is not built."

In receiving the Spingarn Medal, I am proud, humbled, and yes reinvigorated. I believe the awarding of the Spingarn Medal to a scientist for the first time in almost 75 years heralds a new era for Blacks in engineering, medicine, and science in America and indeed the world.

I hope to have your help bringing Black Excellence in Science to even higher levels, because it takes a village.

An important part of my philosophy has been to continue to be appreciative of where I am in life. I have a fortune cookie that sits on my desk that states "If you aren't happy with what you have, how can you be happy with more?"

My philosophy has already included remembering those in the past who helped bring me where I am, proverbially remembering where you came from. Finally, I am a big believer in helping those coming after me. I'm proud to be the first individual to receive all of our nation's highest awards for mentoring: the American Association for the Advancement of Science's Mentor Award, the Beckman Award for Mentoring, and the Presidential Award for Excellence in Science, Math, and Engineering Mentoring bestowed upon me by President Barack Obama.

As the first engineer in history, the fourth physician, and the fifth scientist to receive the Spingarn Medal, I believe I have a tremendous honor, and responsibility, to make a difference in the lives of Black people pursuing scientific professions.

Build Your Spiritual Armor

Make no mistake about it, I am a man who has built his career on science backed by evidence. But above that I am a man who holds his faith greatly. I believe that building the spiritual armor that keeps me going starts with faith. The words of Dr. Martin Luther King, Jr. remind us that "Faith is taking the first step even when you don't see the whole staircase."

I remember that phrase every time I run up multiple flights of stairs. There is an inherent faith that kicks in, as one rounds the corner that more stairs will be there. Faith in the Lord helps us to combat the fear that always takes place in making progress. Faith builds courage, and courage builds hope. Dr. King also stated, "We must build dikes of courage to hold back the flood of fear." Our spiritual armor is the dike of courage.

Each morning when I wake, I first thank God for giving me another day. Nex,t I say the same daily Morning Prayer:

"I am Blessed and Highly Favored. I live in a state of God's holy Grace.

Today, I will Experience God's Grace, Favor and Mercy.

Today, with God's Help, I will reap the Goodness that I have sown. My God is an Awesome God."

I then say something that has stuck with me from an early age, watching television. I say: "Time to Make the Donuts."

The line is from a popular commercial from the 1980s (I think), where the person reflects on his singular and important purpose. It reminds me that whatever I do that day may have profound effects on me and others around me.

I am deeply religious, but I know others may not be. The great thing about God is that you don't have to be. He will meet you wherever you are. I was in Augusta, Georgia, walking. Yes, I am a walking man. I went by a fitness place and took a picture of a verse from the bible that I believe is important (Fig. 2.15).

The verse sums it up. There is Love, Faith, and Hope. Love of God is ideal, Faith in God is wonderful, but just hoping in God's Grace and Mercy provides strength.

Yes, hope is all you need.

Be Fit

A wise man (me) once said:

All the Change You Want to See Begins with You.

I'm a great believer in physical fitness. It is a key to success. The good news is that it doesn't take a lot to be physically fit. In Connecticut, I started the Just Us Moving Program (JUMP Program). The program has at its core, walking for 25 to 45 minutes per day. I started it for a few reasons. First Black, Indigenous, and People of Color often dwell in areas where it is difficult to be physically fit. I've coined the term Exercise Deserts to describe areas where there aren't gyms and/or spas to be physically fit. Walking programs can make the difference. We know at my Institute that our JUMP program not only

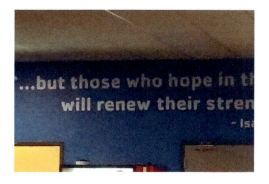

FIGURE 2.15 Those Who Hope

makes people feel better and not only makes people more fit, but our studies are now showing that the 45-minute level of walking each days can help people stave off or manage diabetes. Second, we called it the JUMP program because we know that groups of people walking around together may attract consternation. With tee shirts that say JUMP, those who participate can say, "Hey, it's just us moving!" Third, there is a certain level of health equity that takes place when people can exercise in areas of Exercise Deserts.

That equity can be seen as a form of much needed social justice. Thus, there is a double entendre in the phrase Just Us Moving Program with Justice Moving Program.

The Three A's

The three A's are ability, affability, and availability. They are basic and essential for success. Those that have mastered the three A's have a unique ability to manage their lives and to manage people around them. I emphasize the three A's to my students all the time.

There are some important points to remember about the three A's. The first is, which of the three A's is most important. Most of the time, my students will shout "Ability! Of course!" As it turns out, availability is the most important of the traits to have. Availability is just that, being available. It is a mantra, a way of life that is followed. Great people are greatly available. You send them an email, and you quickly receive an email back. (The email back may not be a long one... it doesn't have to be when someone is super available). A phone call that is made to them garners a quick response by call, text, or email.

Dr Robert Langer is someone that epitomizes the principal of availability. At his 70th birthday celebration, I recounted the story of how I gave Bob a call to ask for some advice. As always, he quickly responded within two rings of the call to his cell. I noticed there seemed to be a speech being made in the background of the call.

"Hello Cato how are you?" he said. "Great Bob, but what's that in the background?" I asked.

"I'm about to get the Wolf Prize, the Israeli Nobel Prize," Bob said in a matter of fact way.

"That's Shimon Perez in the background introducing me."

Apparently I had reached Bob as he was about to come onto the stage to receive one of the world's most prestigious prizes, the Wolf Prize. He was backstage and would soon come be welcomed with tremendous applause. I thought his speaking to me now was extraordinary, even for Bob.

"He is a world leader in science, technology, medicine..." This is what I heard in the background. Shimon Perez was a distinctive orator, and he was in excellent form.

"Bob, Bob... I'll call you back," I'll call you back. Bob at that point was moving closer to the stage and so whispered back. "No don't worry it's a long introduction he's doing on me."

"Let's talk now."

I've learned a lot of lessons from Dr. Langer. Availability is one of them. Availability brings new opportunities. Availability also allows you to take on challenges early on. People who are available appear to others to have it all together, and most of the time they really do.

In this day and age, it's easy to be available. I like to use email. First a word about my philosophy on emails: (1) Emails are for happy thoughts. I never send an email if I am unhappy, or angry. I never send an unhappy email under any circumstances. Yes, there are times when one must communicate unhappiness. Bad news should be given directly, and not by email. (2) Emails should be treated as nonconfidential. My maxim is "A Smile is better than a wink, a wink is better than a nod, a nod is better than a phone call, and everything is better than email." The corollary to that is that nothing should be placed in an email that couldn't be shown on a billboard. (3) Long emails are never needed. Most of my emails are short, they communicate the needed information. In the world of availability, they can be a just a few words. The faster the response, the shorter the email reply needs to be. (4) Always strive to make people feel in a better place with your email. Maya Angelou said, "At the end of the day people won't remember what you said or did, they will remember how you made them feel." An email, however short, can profoundly affect people positively. I am never afraid to provide a word of encouragement or praise, however short in an email.

Being available allows one to take advantage of opportunities. And opportunities can turn into triumphs. Be available, successful people are.

Affability is the second most important key to success. Affability can be defined as being easy to approach and to talk to, friendly, cordial, warmly polite, and showing warmth and friendliness. Many who are affable have a constant optimism about life. The Dalai Lama says, "Be optimistic, it feels better." For many of us though, constantly being optimistic does not come easy. I believe my affability comes from being hopeful about life, and hopeful about the future. It comes from my belief in the greatness of our Lord, and the guiding strength of the Lord. My favorite passage from the Bible is Isaiah 40:31 31. "But those who hope in the LORD will renew their strength. They will soar on wings like eagles; they will run and not grow weary, they will walk and not be faint." My affability, I think comes from my hope for the future, and my belief in God and God's guidance. Desmond Tutu once said, "I am not optimistic, no... I'm quite different from that; I am hopeful. I am a prisoner of hope." Be positive, be affable, and have positive hope for the future.

Ability is the third most important key to success. Cultivating your abilities, developing them to the fullest is keenly important. I am a big fan of Zora Neal Hurston. She was an anthropologist, a writer and filmmaker who was born in the Jim Crow South. She died, the year after I was born, but I still feel a connectedness with her. There are three quotes of Zora Neal Hurston that I strongly relate to. The first is "In the helter-skelter skirmish that is my life,

I have seen that the world is to the strong." Hurston's life was full of highs and lows. But she was someone of tremendous ability who constantly cultivated her knowledge.

The second quote of Hurston's that I admire is "If you are silent about your pain, they'll kill you and say you enjoyed it." It demonstrates a high emotional quotient, which is just as important as "book learning" ability. The third quote is part of the first. Zora Neal Hurston states, "No, I do not weep at the world—I am too busy sharpening my oyster knife." It sums up the three A's. It conveys a sense of urgency and movement to the next level. It conveys a general affability borne of constant hope. And finally, it conveys a constant desire to be sharp and to be able.

The three A's are part of the basics for success in life.

Remember My Lessons to Young People

I often give inspirational speeches to young people about life and what to expect.

They are mainly inspirational, but they provide real truths about the realities of life. I will share one of my typical speeches I've given here. It was at the 2019 Connecticut Invention Competition:

"First let me say how truly honored I feel to be before you today. The Connecticut Invention Convention is a wonderful one, with a long and proud history. You are part of the ranks of the true achievers. Today is a day not of competition ... well maybe it is... but it is absolutely a day to celebrate you, the students who are at this convention. As you continue your road, I would like you to reflect on a few points.

First, I'd like to quote Dean Kamen, the father of the FIRST Robotics program. I first met him in London at a small dinner held on the Future of Engineering."

A Dean Kamen quote is:

"You have teenagers thinking they're going to make millions as NBA stars when that's not realistic for even 1% of them. Becoming a scientist or engineer is."

Dean Kamen's right, and you know that ... you all "get it", by being here, today. Butwhat's more, scientists and engineers really make contributions that change the world and that's really, really important. But, there's also another side. Now I'm from Philadelphia, and there was a song during that period called "Ain't nothing going on but the rent" has anyone heard it ... it's about a woman and a man, well ... let me just tell you the point. The point is that money is important. And what you're doing, puts you on the right track for that, too.

You are living in great times. Challenging times, yes, but challenging times can bring great rewards. If you want to have wealth, *this* is what you should be doing. (Now, I distinguish being rich from having wealth. Being rich means owning two Mercedes, having wealth is being Mercedes.) Again, wealth in this great country called the United States of America is obtained through struggle and seizing opportunities, and those opportunities are often in science and engineering. And many of the people who seized those opportunities started thinking about it at your age.

Take Dean Kamen, for instance, he owns his own island, his own Island (I've not been invited yet, and I'll let you know what that's about after I've visited). Dean Kamen's net worth is thought to be in the Billions … Billions, now that's wealth.

What are some of the key's I can impart you with? First, Education is the key. Dean Kamen says,

" I think an education is not only important, it is the most important thing you can do with your life."

And he's right, So stay in school, and stay in school as long as you can. I got anMD, and a PhD … it was the greatest time of my life. Check that. It was the second greatest time of my life. The greatest time of my life, of course, was meeting, marrying, and being with my wife … but the point is that it's a great time. Enjoy getting smart, and staying smart and get all the education that you can.

Another key for success is:

Being bold, and taking chances in your life. So be bold and take chances. Now, I'm not talking about taking crazy chances like jumping over the Grand Canyon, but measured chances in your life. A common theme for those who are successful is that they took chances. My good friend Mr. Curtis Robinson, a millionaire here in Hartford once said "95% of people don't take chances," and the other 5% own everything.

I want you to take chances, even if they make you uncomfortable. And know that the chances you take may not always go well. My favorite saying is a Zimbabwe African Proverb. "To stumble is not to fall, but to walk faster." (Think about it.) Dr. Martin Luther King Jr said that the ultimate measure of a man is not where he stands in moments of comfort and convenience but where he stands at times of challenge and controversy. Get comfortable being uncomfortable, and get comfortable being on the cutting edge.

I'm going to ask you to do some other things for me. First, as you take on life, remember to enjoy yourself. It's the journey, not the destination that counts. Every day we live is truly a gift for each of us. That's why it's called the present.

Now how do you enjoy the present? Well, as T.I. would say, from his song with Rihanna "Live Your Life" (how many know what I'm talking about), "Stop looking at what you don't have, and start being thankful for what you do have."

Well, what other philosophy can I provide? As you go through the journey, remember a couple of other important things. Build what I call your spiritual armor. Pray, meditate, and hang out with like-minded people, and do so in bad times, but also in good times.

Have Faith. What is Faith? Faith is taking the first step even when you don't see the whole staircase. That's what Martin Luther King said.

The other philosophy point is to find mentors. Look to successful people as role models for you to be successful. You'll find many of these role models share elements of my same philosophy.

I'm really happy for all of you. I'm friends with the singing group Earth Wind and Fire who sang (I know, it's before your time), you're a shining star, no matter who you are, shining bright to see, what you can truly be.

You are all stars, you really are. Remember that. Remember to cherish each day.Take on challenges as opportunities, and build your spiritual armor. And finally, look to others who have gone before you and who are older for inspiration and guidance.

My final thought is that life isn't simple, and it sure isn't easy, in fact life is tough. Think about it, it's so tough, nobody has survived it. The other thing is that I don't think life gets easier, and I'm sorry Dr. Nair, I know this was supposed to be an inspirational message, but it doesn't get easier.

But you get better ... and that's my final message. Life doesn't get easier but you get better.

It's been a really wonderful opportunity, and a privilege to address you. "Good luck today, and throughout your lives. Thanks."

Keep Your Mind Right

I think that attitude is important, always. I teach people to always have a victor mentality and never have a victim mentality. I teach that tough times go away, but tough people don't. I tell people not to dwell in the past—they should have done or could have done. "Don't look back, you're not going that way." I saw a sign once and that stuck with me. Success is about constantly keeping your eyes on the prize, looking through the windshield for what's to come, and not looking through the rear-view mirror, that not how we drive. Most importantly, I teach that you should look toward the end, at the beginning. See things the way you would like things to turn out to be. You have a better chance of having the outcome you want.

I think that perseverance can never be overrated. I believe that success is perseverance for one second more than you need to. To have that kind of success, one must cultivate mental toughness. "The tougher times don't get tougher, but tougher people do." I've discussed the fact that life is about triumphs, opportunities, challenges, and trials. The greatest growth takes place in dealing with challenges in life. The bigger the challenges, the greater the opportunities and success you will see.

Trials can take place in life. The wise Winston Churchill once said, "If You're Going Through Hell ... Keep Going." Remember that the ultimate success is never letting misery have the last word. Trials can include stumbles. It is important to know that stumbles are not a bad thing.

Love More/Save More

I want to make sure there are two important points that I cover. Finding a good partner in life is an important key to success, for a number of reasons. The most important reason is for your sanity. In a study of the University of Tokyo, rats were first given an electric shock. The scientists measured high stress hormone levels in the rats. In a similar study, rats were placed with companion rats (that were not shocked). When the rats were shocked, they had lower stress levels. The take-home message was that in the presence of a companion, stress levels were lower than without a companion. I have mentioned this but want to mention it again. My spouse is a godsend. Now there is science reinforcing the importance of relationships in decreasing stress.

One area crucial to success that is not discussed is that of finances. Gwen Guthrie sings a famous song recorded in the mid-1980s entitled "There's Nothing Goin' on but the Rent." It was a big hit in Philadelphia, where I am from. Debt and overextension are true threats to success. Never live above your means. As much as possible live below your means.

How does one do that? The answer is if you save each week, you will never go into debt. All budgets should include a weekly amount of savings. While money is important, one should never make career moves primarily based on money. If you follow these simple rules, you will be successful financially and in life.

References

1. Wikipedia contributors. *Sea Change (Idiom)*. Wikipedia; December 5, 2019. https://en. wikipedia.org/wiki/Sea_change_(idiom).
2. Blessington M. *America's Sea Change on Racism*. Medium; June 23, 2020. https://medium. com/@mark.blessington/americas-sea-change-on-racism- 19358416c010.
3. Laurencin CT. Diversity 5.0: a way forward. *Journal of Racial and Ethnic Health Disparities*; June 4, 2014. https://link.springer.com/article/10.1007/s40615- 014-0023-5? error=cookies_not_supported&code=4c0ab6b0-4a73-4dc5-b683- 784739f07317.
4. Laurencin CT. *The Context of Diversity*. Science; November 22, 2019. https://science. sciencemag.org/content/366/6468/929.abstract.
5. Laurencin CT. Racial profiling is a public health and health disparities issue. *Journal of Racial and Ethnic Health Disparities*; April 6, 2020. https://link.springer.com/article/10.1007/s40615- 020-00738- 2?error=cookies_not_supported&code=691e670b-47a4-44d6-bbcb-09847af88a53.
6. Laurencin CT. *A Pandemic on a Pandemic: Racism and COVID-19 in Blacks*. PubMed Central (PMC); July 22, 2020. https://www.ncbi.nlm.nih.gov/pmc/articles/PMC7375320/.
7. McClinton A, Laurencin CT. Just in TIME: trauma- informed medical education. *Journal of Racial and Ethnic Health Disparities*; October 1, 2020. https://link.springer.com/article/10. 1007/s40615-020-00881- w?error=cookies_not_supported&code=cb4b3fe8-3dcc-49e1-8e97- f187de306b88.
8. Institute of Medicine (US) Committee on Understanding and Eliminating Racial and Ethnic Disparities in Health Care. *Unequal Treatment: Confronting Racial and Ethnic Disparities in Health Care*. PubMed; 2003. https://pubmed.ncbi.nlm.nih.gov/25032386/.

9. Schneider EC. *Racial Disparities in the Quality of Care for Enrollees in Medicare Managed Care.* PubMed; March 13, 2002. https://pubmed.ncbi.nlm.nih.gov/11886320/.

10. Ryn VM, Burke J. *The Effect of Patient Race and Socio- Economic Status on Physicians' Perceptions of Patients.* PubMed; March 2000. https://pubmed.ncbi.nlm.nih.gov/10695979/.

11. Green A. *Implicit Bias Among Physicians and its Prediction of Thrombolysis Decisions for Black and White Patients.* PubMed Central (PMC); September 1, 2007. www.ncbi.nlm.nih.gov/pmc/articles/PMC2219763/.

12. Barnard G. *["Auction & Negro Sales," Whitehall Street].* The Library of Congress; 1864. https://www.loc.gov/item/2018666988/.

13. American Experience. *Jim Crow Laws.* American Experience | Official Site | PBS; May 16, 2011. https://www.pbs.org/wgbh/americanexperience/features/freedom-riders-jim-crow- laws/.

14. Wang Y. *Workers' or Slaves? Textbook Maker Backtracks after Mother's Online Complaint.* Washington Post; October 5, 2015. https://www.washingtonpost.com/gdpr-consent/?next_ url=https%3a%2f%2fwww.washingtonpost.com%2fnews%2fmorning-mix%2fwp%2f2015% 2f10%2f05%2fimmigrant-workers-or-slaves-textbook-maker-backtracks-after-mothers-online-complaint%2f.

15. Snider MUT. *Kellogg's to Replace Racially Insensitive Corn Pops Boxes Following Twitter Call Out.* USA TODAY; October 26, 2017. https://eu.usatoday.com/story/money/business/2017/10/25/kelloggs-replace- racially-insensitive-corn-pops-boxes-following-twitter-rant/797911001/.

16. Delperdang J. *Check it Out: The Bad Seed & the Good Egg Books by Jory John.* KWIT; October 1, 2019. https://www.kwit.org/post/check-it-out-bad-seed- good-egg-books-jory-john.

17. Jones C. *Levels of Racism: A Theoretic Framework and a Gardener's Tale.* PubMed Central (PMC); August 2000. https://www.ncbi.nlm.nih.gov/pmc/articles/PMC1446334/.

18. Gallagher DABACD. *North Carolina Appeals Court Blocks Voter ID Law - CNNPolitics.* CNN; February 19, 2020. https://edition.cnn.com/2020/02/18/politics/north-carolina-voter-id-law/index.html.

19. Isidore C. *Ally to Pay $98 Million to Settle Car Loan Discrimination Probe.* CNNMoney; December 20, 2013. https://money.cnn.com/2013/12/20/news/companies/ally-car-loan-discrimination/.

20. Reports — CT Racial Profiling Prohibition Project. *CT Racial Profiling Prohibition Project*; May 2016. http://www.ctrp3.org/reports/.

21. Basken P. *NIH Allocates $31-Million to Tackle Racial Gaps in Training.* The Chronicle of Higher Education; October 22, 2014. https://www.chronicle.com/article/nih-allocates-31-million-to-tackle-racial-gaps- in-training/.

22. Ginther DK, Schaffer WT, Schnell J, Masimore B, Liu F, Haak LL, et al. Race, Ethnicity, and NIH Research Awards. Science (New York). 2011; 333(6045):1015—1019. https://doi.org/10.1126/science.1196783. PMID: 21852498; PMCID: PMC3412416

23. White Coats for Black Lives. #BlackLivesMatter: physicians must stand for racial justice. *Journal of Ethics | American Medical Association*; October 1, 2015. https://journalofethics.ama-assn.org/article/blacklivesmatter-physicians-must- stand-racial-justice/2015-10.

24. Wikipedia contributors. *Allostatic Load.* Wikipedia; October 26, 2020. https://en.wikipedia.org/wiki/Allostatic_load#:%7E:text=Allostatic load is %22the wear,McEwen and Stellar in 1993.

25. McEwen BS, Stellar E. *Stress and the Individual. Mechanisms Leading to Disease.* PubMed; September 27, 1993. https://pubmed.ncbi.nlm.nih.gov/8379800/.

26. Orom H, Sharma C, Homish G, Underwood W, Homish D. *Racial Discrimination and Stigma Consciousness Are Associated with Higher Blood Pressure and Hypertension in Minority Men.* PubMed; October 31, 2016. https://pubmed.ncbi.nlm.nih.gov/27800597/.

27. Duru O, Harawa N, Kermah D, Norris K. *Allostatic Load Burden and Racial Disparities in Mortality.* PubMed; August 12, 2012. https://www.ncbi.nlm.nih.gov/pmc/articles/PMC3417124/.

28. Brewer L, Carson K, Williams D, Allen A, Jones C, Cooper L. *Association of Race Consciousness with the Patient–Physician Relationship, Medication Adherence, and Blood Pressure in Urban Primary Care Patients.* PubMed; November 26, 2013. https://www.ncbi.nlm.nih.gov/pmc/articles/PMC3790452/.

29. Laurencin CT, Murdock C, Laurencin L, Christensen D. HIV/AIDS and the African-American community 2018: a decade call to action. *Journal of Racial and Ethnic Health Disparities*; June 4, 2018. https://link.springer.com/article/10.1007/s40615-018-0491- 0?error=cookies_not_supported&code=de5df31c-4792-4aca-9127-7577a8c5060d.

30. Ribaudo H, Smith K, Robbins G, et al. *Racial Differences in Response to Antiretroviral Therapy for HIV Infection: An AIDS Clinical Trials Group (ACTG) Study Analysis.* PubMed; December 1, 2013. https://www.ncbi.nlm.nih.gov/pmc/articles/PMC3814827/.

31. NCHHSTP Media Team. *2016 CROI Press Release: Lifetime HIV Risk | CDC.* CDC; February 23, 2016. https://www.cdc.gov/nchhstp/newsroom/2016/croi-press-release-risk.html.

32. Lee M. *Does the United States Really Have 5 Percent of the World's Population and One Quarter of the World's Prisoners?* The Washington Post; April 30, 2015. https://www.washingtonpost.com/gdpr- consent/?next_url=https%3a%2f%2fwww.washingtonpost.com%2fnews%2ffact-checker%2fwp%2f2015%2f04%2f30%2fdoes-the-united-states-really-have-five- percent-of-worlds-population-and-one-quarter-of-the-worlds-prisoners%2f.

33. Gramlich J. *The Gap between the Number of Blacks and Whites in Prison is Shrinking.* Pew Research Center; April 30, 2019. https://www.pewresearch.org/fact- tank/2019/04/30/shrinking-gap-between-number-of-blacks-and-whites-in-prison/.

34. Badger E, Miller C, Pearce A, Quealy K. *Extensive Data Shows Punishing Reach of Racism for Black Boys.* The New York Times; March 19, 2018. https://www.nytimes.com/interactive/2018/03/19/upshot/race-class-white-and- black-men.html.

35. Tyeese D. *Are Black Male Doctors Becoming Endangered?* The Grio; March 5, 2013. https://thegrio.com/2013/03/05/are-black-male-doctors-becoming- endangered/.

36. Laurencin CT, Murray M. *An American Crisis: The Lack of Black Men in Medicine.* PubMed; June 1, 2018. https://www.ncbi.nlm.nih.gov/pmc/articles/PMC5909952/.

37. Laurencin CT. *An American Crisis: The Growing Absence of Black Men in Medicine and Science: Proceedings of a Joint Workshop.* The National Academies Press; 2018. https://www.nap.edu/read/25130/chapter/1.

38. Gamblin M. *A Reflection on Anti-black Racism.* Bread for the World; August 9, 2020. https://www.bread.org/blog/reflection-anti-black-racism.

39. Wikipedia contributors. *Anti-racism.* Wikipedia; October 22, 2020a. https://en.wikipedia.org/wiki/Anti-racism.

40. Ballestrini C. *U.S. Anti-black Racism Course.* Office of the Provost; October 6, 2020. https://provost.uconn.edu/us-anti-black-racism-course/.

41. Herbert W, Nickens Award. *AAMC*; 2021. https://www.aamc.org/what-we-do/aamc-awards/nickens.

Chapter 3

The Lessons

When you look at my CV and my papers, patents, and accomplishments, what you don't see is the lessons that came from each and every step. By sharing my hard-earned lessons, I hope that some of them will resonate and be helpful to you as you strive for your own success.

1) Know Who You Are. Don't Let Others Define You

Once, when I was the Vice President for Health Affairs at the University of Connecticut, I was sitting in the stadium in the Provost's box watching a football game. A person came over to me to sit down and say hello.

"Hello, I've been told that you are the head of the medical center," she stated.

"Yes," I said. "I'm the Vice President for Health Affairs and the Dean of the Medical School."

"That's extraordinary that someone with your background would be the head of the medical center. I've always thought the head of a medical center would have to be a physician or a dentist, or have some medical background," she said.

Well, yes, I am a physician.

No, you're not.

"Well, thanks," I said, "but I'm am a physician."

No, I know you are not. I was told you played professional football for a number of years and now they made you head of the medical center.

Nope, I never played football.

Yes, you did.

No, I'm sure I didn't. I'm pretty sure I would know. I didn't, really.

She stood up, frustrated with my answers. She turned to walk away, and then turned around again. With one final incredulous look she asked.

Well, if you aren't a former professional football player, running the medical center, why would they all say that you are?

Success Is What You Leave Behind. https://doi.org/10.1016/B978-0-12-417224-1.00003-1

119

In some ways, that was probably the only sane part of the conversation I had with her. Somehow, being a tall Black man, led to the weaving of an incredible story that the University had hired a former professional football player to be the head of the medical center. I guess it was more believable than hiring a Black physician who graduated from Harvard Medical.

Coming from the inner city of Philadelphia through education at Harvard and MIT to numerous jobs as an engineer, physician, and scientist, to the present, I have come across numerous cases of others trying to define me. Some of the time the attempts represent gaslighting.

This wasn't the first time I was mistaken for someone I wasn't. When I was in third-grade school, the counselors told my parents and I that I shouldn't waste my time going to high school. They felt I should enter vocational school instead of an academic high school. They recommended that I become an air-conditioning technician, specifically. They were so sure I would not make it through the rigors of high school. They were sure that would be a good trade for someone like me.

There is little question that many of my experiences of being categorized and boxed in have been clearly racially motivated. It's a reality that Black people face, and it is unfair. That experience is magnified for Blacks, but it isn't a uniquely Black experience. There is a universality that takes place. Parents, teachers, counselors, bosses—all have their own perceptions of who you are and who you should be. And all too often their notions, no matter how well-meaning, can define you as a marginalized version of the person than you are capable of being. Their words can narrow, edit, and shape your own vision of yourself and close you off from your potential. They can shape your life if you let them and if you don't have advocates who are committed to speaking up for you, and to you when you need it.

But how can you keep other people's definitions from constricting you? How do you avoid assimilating the message of your limitations and define yourself according to your own best lights?

That's an obvious challenge for kids growing up in the inner city. It's less obvious but equally challenging for scientists, engineers, doctors, and businessmen of color. So often, even high achievers fail to mobilize their full potential. Much of the talent and creativity they have inside them goes untapped—because they have been conditioned to think of themselves in limited ways. They have internalized the definitions others have laid down for generations. The problem cuts right across the board, from youngsters struggling to find themselves to professionals well along in their careers. What, then, are the keys to unlocking our fullest potential? What resources can we draw on to define ourselves, keep the definitions of others at bay, and pursue the highest level of achievement we are capable of?

First, define yourself. Who are you and what do you stand for, and what do you want to become. Defining yourself goes a long way toward not only building your personal self-esteem, but also in deciding what you need to do to better yourself. Under smart, hardworking, loyal, good person, courageous, adaptable, and resilient (the principal traits for success) how to define yourself and who you are. Once you have a firm grasp on who you are better prepared to take on the world.

Second, understand that there are the people who are speaking to you and about you who are planting false narratives about your potential. In my own life, there have been five types of people who spoke and try to still speak to me and provide input about who I am. There are those who hate, those who are my friends (but are not my friends), those who are critics, and those who are loyal friends/family. Always remember that those who hate you and want to diminish you don't know you and are not there for you. Their opinions of you should be completely discounted.

Those who are friends/but not friends know you, but are not for you. Their opinions should be discounted, but not completely. They have enough knowledge about you that they may understand weaknesses that may be important to address. Critics don't know you and are not for or against you. This is an important group of people to listen to because they "don't have a dog in the fight" as it has been said. Finally, loyal friends/family are people who know you and are for you. They are an important group to listen to. They do have dog in the fight per se, and that fight is for you. Remember there are exceptions to any rule, and goes for audience rules above.

Third, and perhaps most important, there is a certain part of life that one has to be "Ray Charles to the Bull" as first stated by rapper Lil Wayne and paraphrased by me here. The term to me means two things. First, the obvious is that Ray Charles was blind and so turning a "blind eye" to those who would define you in ways that would detract from you should be done. But there is another point to the term in my mind. Ray Charles was the ultimate definer of himself. A poor child growing up in the rural South who becomes blind … it is a story that in his time might have a tragic end. The expectations placed on Ray Charles were low. Yet he defined himself and his capacities. And if you ever followed his journey, you know he worked hard to be a master entertainer constantly redefined and improved himself, despite the hurdles and haters around him. To me, he epitomizes the lesson: "Know Who You Are. Don't Let Others Define You."

2) Walk with People Smarter Than You

This is a phrase from my grandmother, Madge McIntosh Morehead, who with my grandfather, Hosea Morehead, were the cornerstones of our family. That lesson was passed on to my mother, who passed it on to us, her children. One of my sisters put her own twist on it. "You can't fly high," she says, "if you're hanging with turkeys."

My life has been about seeking out and aligning with people who are smarter than I am. I grow and gain energy from them.

When I made my acceptance remarks for winning the Spingarn Medal, the highest honor of the NAACP, they reflected and still underscore my philosophy of the value of being surrounded by people who smarter than me.

"I want to first begin by thanking the leadership of the NAACP, especially the Spingarn Award Committee, for selecting me to receive this singular honor which is the Spingarn Medal. I want to thank Dr. Dwayne Proctor, Chair of the NAACP Foundation, and Mr. Scott Esdaile, the President of the Connecticut NAACP, my brothers in arms, for their friendship and support.

"I want to thank the great Professor Robert Langer, a chemical engineer, and my mentor. I want to thank and pay tribute to Dr. Louis Sullivan who introduced me. He is a tremendous physician—scientist and administrator who has helped pave the way for me and many others. Dr. Langer and Dr. Sullivan, I appreciate both of you.

The list of those who have won the Spingarn Medal is incredible and includes Dr. Martin Luther King, Jr, George Washington Carver, Ernest Just, Percy Julian, and the great Maya Angelou. I am honored to be in such awesome company.

I want to pay homage to those who have come before me. Maya Angelou wrote, "I am a Black Ocean, leaping and wide. Welling and swelling I bear in the tide. Bringing the gifts that my ancestors gave. I am the dream and the hope of the slave. I rise. I rise, I rise."

From Cato, who led the Cato Rebellion in South Carolina in 1741, to Cato Wilson, born in Georgia in 1811, to Cato Wilson, my namesake, a class of 1895 graduate of Meharry Medical College, thank you. Thank you for your persistence, your perseverance, and your determination.

I want to thank my father Cyril Laurencin, a strong union carpenter, and my mother Dr. Helen I. Moorehead Laurencin, a trailblazer in medicine and science and a leader of her community in North Philadelphia.

My parents taught me Black Excellence. My parents taught me Black Resilience. Because of them, to paraphrase Drizzy Drake, "I'm on a roll like Cottenelle, because I was made for all this stuff."

Moving now to the present, I pay homage to my wife Cynthia and my beautiful and intelligent children. Thank you, I love you, you motivate me each day to strive. And to my many colleagues and students, I share this day, and this award with you.

I had the honor of winning Africa's Science Prize, the UNESCO Equatorial Guinea International Prize for Research in the Life Sciences. I shared it with among others, Tu Youyou, the first woman from China to win the Nobel Prize. I am the first person from the African diaspora to receive this award. When I addressed the leaders of the African Union last year in Ethiopia, I stated that we need to create new initiatives uniting Black people throughout the world in the pursuit of engineering, medicine, and science. A daunting task yes, but there is a Massai proverb that states, "The village which is not discussed is not built."

In receiving the Spingarn Medal, I am proud, humbled, and yes rein-vigorated. I believe the awarding of the Spingarn Medal to a scientist for the first time in almost 75 years heralds a new era for Blacks in engineering, medicine, and science in America and indeed the world.

I hope to have your help bringing Black Excellence in Science to even higher levels, because it takes a village.

Thank you again for this tremendous honor."

3) Making Moves to Surround Myself with Excellence

When I was in the fourth grade, my parents moved me from a seriously underachieving neighborhood school to a Catholic school. After that, they sent me to Philadelphia's elite academic high school. At St. Stephen's Catholic School, I was drawn by the friendship of the smartest kid in the class. At Central High School, a teacher told me he was putting me in an AP class. I had never heard of AP, but the students there seemed unusually intelligent. When I was ready for college, I was wowed by a recruiting team from Princeton's School of Engineering that was visiting Philadelphia high schools, even though I had no intention of becoming an engineer. The dinner program I attended for Princeton engineering was at the Four Seasons hotel. As an inner-city high school kid, I didn't get out much. The Four Season facility was spectacular and the ambiance added to the special occasion. The Princeton faculty member who sat at my table was incredibly smart, but also witty and engaging. At the end of the dinner, the moderator for the evening introduced the speaker. After an impressive introduction and loud applause, I was surprised to see the faculty member I engaged with all evening rise. He was the keynote speaker. He gave a talk equal to his great reputation.

By the time I completed my 4 years at Princeton, as a chemical engineer, I had internalized the principle. If you want to push yourself to the maximum, walk with the smartest. Associate yourself with the best people you can find, who are doing the things you want to do, whether you're a scientist or a carpenter or whatever else you might be. Put yourself in their path, in their penumbra. Watch what they do and how they do it—and why they do it. When you see people who are smarter than you are, who are the smartest people around, that's who you go with, that's whom you hitch your wagon to.

When I started at Harvard Medical School, I was determined enough to ask: Who's the smartest person here? I want him to be my advisor." Imagine if you were interested in computer programming 15 years ago and had hung round with Mark Zuckerberg.

When asked about the life lessons he's learned, one of the greatest athletes to ever play basketball and stellar businessman, Earvin "Magic" Johnson, said the first one that came to mind was "Always Run with the Best." He said he had learned that from Michael Jordan. "There's nothing like it for lifting your game," Johnson said. I understand that and live by it.

Getting back to Harvard Medical School, my grandmother's message resonated as I walked inside the ivy-laden buildings. I met my first advisor, an award-winning hematologist. I immediately began with "I want to be with the smartest person at Harvard. Are you the smartest person?" He smiled and then chuckled. He said there were so many smart people to choose from, I didn't need to find the smartest person. My attitude was a bit different at the time. Yes, I was at Harvard. If I could identify the smartest person in an environment of extremely bright people, that person could serve as a superadvisor. At the end of the conversation, he taciturnly stated "No, I don't know who the smartest person is, I certainly am not."

During the year, I continued to meet many brilliant individuals at Harvard. The ones I was most impressed with I asked, "Are you the smartest person at Harvard?" Invariably, the answer was no, I am not the smartest person. I would quickly thank the person, and move on. By the time I was two-thirds of the way through the year, I had not found the smartest person. Indefatigable though, I heard a lecture in pathophysiology that was fascinating, and it featured the research of a bright young faculty member. At the end of the class, I approached him regarding the smartest person at Harvard. He began to state what I had heard all year, but this time with a twist. He said, he was not the smartest person, but he thought he knew who was.

The person's name was Dr. Judah Folkman.

Dr. Folkman was a towering figure in medicine and science. A board-certified pediatric surgeon. And he was also a trailblazing researcher in the area of angiogenesis and antiangiogenesis. I immediately called and made an appointment to meet with him. I came to his office at Boston Children's Hospital. His clinical office adjoined his laboratory. I sat down and said, "Dr. Folkman, I've heard you are the smartest person at Harvard. I want to be with the smartest person here. Are you the smartest person at Harvard?" Without missing a beat, Dr. Folkman said "Yes, I am." I then replied, "Well alright!" And the rest was history. He became an important advisor for me and as I discuss in a later lesson an important source of my philosophy of life.

Fast forwarding from the end of my first year at Harvard to my third year, I began work in the laboratory of the great Professor Robert Langer. One day, Bob came by my desk and said he wanted me to meet the smartest person at Harvard. I told him that I would be very glad to meet someone that he regarded as the smartest person at Harvard, but I already know the smartest person at Harvard and have known him for 2 years. As I walked into Bob Langer's office, my philosophy came full circle. In Bob Langer's office was Dr. Judah Folkman. It turns out that Bob Langer sought him out in much the same way I did a number of years before and became an advisee of Dr. Folkman. We all laughed and then all agreed we had indeed found the smartest person at Harvard. The episode reinforced the lesson of Walking With People Smarter Than You. Truly successful people like Dr. Langer use this principle in their work and interactions as well.

This is a principle that is just as important when you build your teams throughout your career.

4) Do an Adhimu Chunga

Adhimu Chunga was a Princeton upperclassman when I arrived as a freshman. His real name was Larry Hamm, but Adhimu Chunga was his nom de struggle. He was from Newark, New Jersey. Adhimu was the head of the Black Students Association. In 1973, the New York Times wrote a profile on him, Adhimu Chunga, 19 and Angry. He was profiled because, at 19, he was the youngest and most controversial member of the Newark School Board. He would go on to run for US Senator against Senator Corey Booker.

The year after I arrived at Princeton, Adhimu Chunga, and the Black Students Association decided to stage a rolling social justice campaign. It was a great and ambitious idea. They would start in South Jersey and make their way north, stopping at courthouses and city halls to hold rallies and mobilize support for affordable housing, early enrichment programs, and help for women and children.

During my time at Princeton, I was involved with student politics. I was one of the few Blacks that worked in the mainstream political spheres (Undergraduate Student Government (USG) and University Council (U-Council)) and at the same time was involved with the National Society of Black Engineers (NSBE). I had heard some of the background on the plan and had decided to come and hear the whole plan and see if I could help. I RSVP's for the first meeting.

I was impressed by Adhimu Chunga. I took home a lot of lessons that day. First, he was prepared, really prepared. He knew everyone by name, even me. Now that might not seem very impressive, but I had never met him, and he knew my name. Second, he knew everyone's expertise. He knew I was an engineer. At the same time, he knew that I worked in Student Government. In fact, that was why I was invited. He had done his homework.

As we sat around the event committee table, Adhimu asked me not be shy and to take a seat around the table near him. Then he laid out the events of the planned March with surgical precision. Finally, he issued a budget. Ninety percent of the budget was one item, the buses that would transport people to and from the event. The cost was $10,000.

To put this in perspective, this was $10,000 in 1970s money. This was a huge amount. But the plan called for it. Buses had to be available on demand for an entire day. The logistics of food, advertisement all called for funding. But the buses were the biggest cost.

Adhimu Chunga's turned to me with a determined look. I had to deliver 20 buses on the day of the rally. This was my assignment. The cost for this was $10,000.

The only way I could think to get that sum was to ask the Undergraduate Student Government. There was a fund for organizations doing activities. But they told me there were 150 student organizations, and the budget was divided among them. The Black Students Association would receive its share and no more, which was a very small part of the amount I needed. I had made some behind the scenes inquiries and found the budget for all activities for the year was approximately $30,000. I could hope at best to get $300 for the Black Students Association.

At our next event meeting, Adhimu went around the table, getting reports from the communications person, the PR person, the water and food person, and so on. And then it came me. I told him what those at Undergraduate Student Government relayed to me. I told him that there were no ways I could think of to raise that level of money.

"I want you to re-think your thinking," he said. "I want you to find a way. Always think that there is a way. It may be hard, but there is a way," he added with absolute determination. "Your assignment is to get those buses."

Our next meeting would be 3 weeks from that day. "As we go around the room—and this goes for all in the room—my expectation is that you state succinctly that all is set," he said and he meant it. And because he was so sure and had entrusted me with delivering on that trust, I knew what I had to do.

I went back to the Undergraduate Student Government. I made a passionate request for us to do something differently this year as students. Instead of funding 10 dollars here or $100 there, to pick one big humanitarian event for once that would benefit not just the students but also people in the community. They agreed and voted for the first time to provide a large chunk of the student activities budget for the Black Students Association event. They provided $10,000 to be precise, to pay for buses.

At our next event meeting, all the leaders assigned with tasks sat at the table. Chunga rattled off the assignments and people succinctly replied. "Food?" Ordered. Public Relations? All in place. Buses? Buses will be there. Medical! EMTs alerted. Banners! Complete." "OK, alright, we are set." Then he turned to me and provided a quick knowing nod that I will never forget. He then turned to the rest of the table and shouted, "Meeting adjourned!"

Watching him in action was a transformational experience. Chunga had challenged me to do something I thought was truly impossible and I had done it. When that kind of thing happens to you, it changes your life. If you take the task on, it forces you to challenge your creativity, your intelligence, and your skill. And if you're successful, it gives an explosive shock to the way you see yourself. From here on in you know, you're capable of doing things you couldn't have imagined doing before. It stretches your limits and opens you up to your own possibilities. Again, as Bob Marley states, "You never know how strong you are, until being strong is your only choice." Adhimu has fought the good fight of activism for 50 years and is still going strong.

To this day, at my Institute at the University of Connecticut, when I say "We need to do an Adhimu Chunga," everyone knows what I mean. Having an Adhimu Chunga mindset infuses the group with a sense of possibility. We know we need to do something that at first glance might not seem possible. But we're primed to do it because we've done it before. Doing an Adhimu Chunga boosts the potential of an individual and an organization. It's also the most powerful mechanism for personal growth there is.

5) To Stumble Isn't to Fall, but to Walk Faster

This is a Zimbabwe proverb. It tells you that when you stumble what happens is that you try to catch yourself, and when you do you actually gain speed. In life too, a stumble can force you to move faster. Things that are in your way, which seem like obstacles, often give you an unexpected chance to light a fire under your work and your career.

I've had more stumbles than I can count. Most of us have. One big one for me happened when I had just finished my MD and my graduate work. I had started up my lab at MIT and I was beginning an internship in Philadelphia's Pennsylvania Hospital. Every day I talked by phone with my graduate student lab assistant, and every weekend, I went rushing back to Boston to work on our experiments.

One day, I called Bob Langer from Philadelphia just to check in. He was my mentor, and I talked with him regularly. He wasn't in, but his assistant was. "How's everything going?" I asked.

"Fine," she said, "except that they just closed the department."

"Don't joke like that," I said.

"I'm not joking," she said. "They've closed the department."

MIT had indeed decided to close the Department of Applied Biological Sciences and move the professors to other more traditional departments. Langer was going to chemical engineering, others to neuroscience and elsewhere. It wasn't clear where I was going. I was a new instructor with a small start-up lab. And I hadn't seen it coming.

When I signed on, MIT had given me a bare bones start-up budget, scarcely enough to get going. Now that my department was closed, they definitely wouldn't be giving me any more funding or extending themselves in any other way. I needed outside funding and I needed it fast.

I quickly applied to the Whitaker Foundation, a likely source. They funded bioengineering projects and I was proposing to study how to generate bone using synthetic materials, just down their alley, or so I thought.

To my severe disappointment, they sent back a rejection. Undaunted, and remembering the proverb, I reworked the proposal, doubled the budget, and submitted it to the National Science Foundation. I received phenomenal scores for that proposal. I actually received a phone call from the program director praising me on the quality of the grant. My quick decision and my resilience funded my research at a critical time and then put me in a good position to elicit more funding and expand the work I was doing.

What happened? The department closure had kickstarted my search for funding. The Whitaker rejection, another stumble, had forced me to look for something bigger. Understand that not every stumble I've made has worked out for the better. But most have. The significant thing is to get that

Zimbabwean proverb embedded in your head—to be able to see setbacks as potential openings for growth and success.

The Zimbabwe proverb is actually a part of triad of my philosophy.

1. Tough times take place, but, you only fall if you decide to.
2. Stumbling is not falling—Malcolm X.
3. To stumble is not to fall but to walk faster.

Falling is bad. Falling can feel like failure. People have asked me when I have failed, as if all that I have worked for and accomplished always came easy and without struggle. But I can tell them I never have failed. Why? Because failing is something you accept. Failing is something that you must actively participate in. I have never failed. But I have stumbled many times. As Malcolm X taught, there is a big difference between stumbling and failing or falling.

What are the keys to walking faster after a stumble? First, there is a belief in the divine God. My favorite gospel group is Anthony Brown and therAPY. My favorite song is History. The song's lyrics are as follows:

Something good is coming to me
How do I know? 'Cause we got history
Haha, yeah, let's go
Good days and bad days
Each day I still say
Thank You for letting me see it
Some days I still face
Trials and I say
I wish I didn't have to go through this
(I wish)
But that's when I remember Your love
Your love surrounding me, yeah
That's when I remember Your touch
Your hand is holding me, yeah
I know You have tomorrow
Just like You've got today, yeah
Have not forgotten what You did for me yesterday
We still got history
(Yeah, yeah, yeah, we do)
We've got history
(Yeah, yeah, yeah, we do)
We've got history
(Yeah, yeah, yes, we do)
We've got history
Of me praising You and You coming through for me
Oh, oh, oh-oh-oh, oh
And I love our story

Oh, oh, oh-oh-oh, oh
And I love our story
Oh, oh, oh-oh-oh, oh
And I love our story
Oh, oh, oh-oh-oh, oh
And I love our story
Each day Your mercies
You freely give me
Thank You for letting me see it
Yeah, I owe You that much
Even on rough days
'Cause You put a smile on my face
Somehow I know we're gonna get through it
That's 'cause I remember Your love
Your love surrounding me, yeah
That's 'cause I remember Your touch
Your hand is holding me, yeah
I know You have tomorrow
Just like You've got today, yeah
Have not forgotten what You did for me yesterday
'Cause we've got history
(We do, we do, ooh)
We've got history
(We do, we do, ooh)
We've got history
(We do, we do, ooh)
We've got history
Of me praising You and You coming
Oh, oh, oh-oh-oh, oh
And I love our story
Oh, oh, oh-oh-oh, oh
And I love our story
Oh, oh, oh-oh-oh, oh
And I love our story
Oh, oh, oh-oh-oh, oh
God, I love our story
You have not been given the spirit of fear
But the power of love and a sound mind
So before I start worrying
I ask myself this one question
Why would He not show up again
When He showed up the last time?
Didn't He show up the last time?
Yeah, He showed up the last time

Why would He not show up again
When He showed up the last time?
Didn't He show up the last time?
Yeah, He showed up the last time
Why would He not heal me again
When He healed me the last time?
Didn't He heal me the last time?
Yeah, He healed me the last time
Why would He not heal me again
When He healed me the last time?
Didn't He heal me the last time?
Yeah, He healed me the last time
Why would He not keep me again
When He kept me the last time?
Didn't He keep me the last time?
Yeah, He kept me the last time
Why would He not keep me again
When He kept me the last time?
Didn't He keep me the last time?
Yeah, He kept me the last time
Why would He not show up again?
Why would He not show up again?
Why would He not show up again?
Why would He not show up again?
I know You have tomorrow
Just like You've got today, yeah
I have not forgotten what You did for me yesterday.
I know You have tomorrow
Just like You've got today, yeah
I have not forgotten what You did for me yesterday
I know You have tomorrow
Just like You've got today, yeah
I have not forgotten what You did for me yesterday
'Cause we've got history
(I remember, yeah)
We've got history
(Mmh, help me to remember that we're got)
We've got history
(Yeah, I'm still praising You off our history)
We've got history
Of me praising You and You coming through for me
Believe in The Lord. Let me say this again. Believe in the Lord. Earlier I
wrote the prayer I say each day I open my eyes and God has blessed me in
providing me another day.

"I am Blessed and Highly Favored.
I live in a state of God's holy Grace.
Today, I will Experience God's Grace, Favor and Mercy.
Today, with God's Help, I will reap the Goodness that I have sown.
My God is an Awesome God."
Count on God. Whether you know it or not, you and he have history.
Otherwise, you would not be here right now.
(Why would he not show up again, didn't he show up the last time?)
Second, understand what life is really about. This is what life is in a
nutshell.
Triumphs, opportunities, challenges, tests, trials, and hard times.
There, I said it.
While we all welcome the triumphs and opportunities, the truth is that we
face more challenges, tests, trials, and hard times. An important Latin phrase is
Per aspera ad astra. It means "through hardships to the stars." I encourage you
to embrace the hardships. They are the true gateway to success.
In January of 2020, I was notified that I had won the Kappa Delta Award. It
had been called the Nobel Prize for Orthopaedic Surgery Research. My
coauthors were Dr. Yusuf Khan and Dr. Lakshmi Nair, two scientists, who
combined have been with me for a total of over 50 years. They started as my
students and now are my colleagues. When I got the award and informed them,
Yusuf Khan sent me a screenshot of the applications we submitted to get the
award. We had applied for the award 21 times! 20 times we experienced the
disappointment of not getting the award. And 20 times we asked ourselves if
we should apply again. But we all understood what life is really about. And we
were undaunted. We applied again.
I find that one of the things that hold people back is not understanding how
stumbling can be a good thing. I have sat on a number of awards committee
and have seen people who are the number two person for an award, who would
have surely gotten the award the next year, not apply for the award the next
year after being rejected. What a shame. The intervening year allowed for
people on the committee to digest and understand more about them and why
they should be number one. They would have surely gotten the award.
Stumbling is not falling, but walking faster, but it is up to you to take
advantage of this wisdom.
You have to be prepared for life. Earlier I wrote about the fact that Life is
tough. Life is so tough, that, really, no one has survived it. But over time, life,
even as it gets tougher, you can manage it. Life gets tougher, but you get better.
You get better through PREParation. PREP as I have called it is persistence, resilience, emotional quotient, and perseverance. I will discuss them out
of order as they make more sense. Think of yourself on a boat traveling on
rough seas. Persistence is that quality that allows you to keep moving in seas,
even when they are rough. Perseverance is that quality that allows you to keep
moving in the rough seas, even as you are buffeted, almost falling from the

boat. Resilience is the quality that allows you to get back into the boat after the water has been so strong it has knocked you out of the boat. Emotional Quotient is the quality that allows you to decide to take the trip in the unstable waters in the first place.

Stumbling can work to your advantage only if you have built your PREP. By doing this, you can make stumbling event occasions where you walk faster and succeed.

6) If You Can Walk, You Can Dance; If You Can Talk, You Can Sing

This is another Zimbabwean Proverb. This one has to do with finding out how to push your talents. The great American psychologist William James maintained that we use "only a small part of our possible mental and physical resources." When I talk to youngsters, I usually give it a more proactive twist. "What you don't know about our capabilities," I tell them, "is far greater than what you do know." That's true for almost all of us.

What's the secret of people whose accomplishments seem extraordinary? Is it simply talent, or intelligence, or is there something even more fundamental at work? What gives a person the desire and drive to explore how far they might be able to go?

Working to capacity is a big part of leading a fulfilled life. But the first step is wanting to explore what that capacity is. You have to be aware you can push the envelope before you do push the envelope. So, what can you do to open your mind to your own possibilities? And what can you do as a mentor and leader to inspire others to do the same?

COVID 19 reinforced this for me. It was bad. I was at home, watching NETFLIX, like everyone was. My research laboratory was shut down, and frankly I was very down.

I called my mentor Dr. Langer. In the background I heard a whirl of an elliptical machine and rush of weights he was wielding in his hands. "I have to tell you this is the best time for me. It has really tested me and I have had to move to the next level," he said. He then told me everything he was doing from the new science in his lab, to developing a vaccine to end the COVID pandemic. It was extraordinary, but it was so "BOB." Dr. Langer was one of the founders of Moderna. Besides inventing the technology that would save the world, he became an overnight multibillionaire. He is, if you don't know it from my book so far, MY HERO.

The call with him was invigorating and transformative. I gathered my team together and said we will spend the year writing up our research, writing up review papers. The group responded, and we had our best year in terms of production of papers and patents. At the same time, I was inspired to do my part to fight the COVID epidemic. I and my team wrote the first paper in the refereed literature on Blacks and COVID-19. I became an advocate on making sure people in Connecticut and indeed nation-wide understood COVID 19, what it was about and how deadly it was, especially to the communities of color. I was proud to be named a Connecticut Healthcare Hero by Connecticut Magazine for my work in publishing the first data on COVID-19 in America.

Overall, my call to the team yielded incredible results. Not only were we in the forefront on COVID 19 in communities of color, we published a piece describing a newer, safer way to greet each other during the pandemic. The greeting became known as the Laurencin-McClinton greeting. Dr. McClinton is an incredibly gifted surgeon who was my fellow for a year.

"In the time of a pandemic, societies adopt practices that necessitate the least human contact. To curtail the spread of coronavirus disease 2019 (COVID-19), people have transitioned to social distancing and replaced gestures of greeting and parting for an alternative acknowledgment. In the early days of the pandemic, people were waving, bowing, foot tapping, and elbow bumping. It is difficult to predict how COVID-19 will reshape social etiquette. Perhaps alternative greetings will define a new normal for social interaction.

In "normal" times, the handshake transcends culture and geographic boundaries. Its origin is found in ancient Greek history as a gesture representing an offering of peace. In modern times, it symbolizes greeting, establishes respect, offers congratulations, and solidifies farewell.

Although hand hygiene is a recommended guideline for infection control, its practice is variable. Healthcare providers maintain an average adherence rate of only 40%. A study that directly observed hand washing after restroom use found that 67% of individuals used soap when washing their hands, 10% did not wash their hands at all, and only 5% washed their hands for the recommended duration. A handshake can transfer 124 million bacteria, twice as many pathogens as a high five. Contamination is associated with the area of contact, and the largest contact area is obtained with a handshake. We may benefit from avoiding hand contact altogether.

The pandemic has inspired creative alternatives. Some advocate for noncontact greetings such as a wave or customary bowing. A study concluded that within the healthcare setting, 78% of patients prefer that their physician greets them with a handshake. The foot tap involves individuals tapping their feet together to greet. The elbow bump may be less than ideal considering that some societies advocate for people to sneeze and cough into their elbow.

The fist bump transmits the lowest number of pathogens in comparison with a handshake and high five. Among volunteers on a surgical ward, the colonization of the palmar surface of the hand after a handshake was four times greater than that of the fist after a fist bump. The fist bump is derived from dap, a language of gestures rooted in Black American history. It emerged in the 1960s among Black soldiers during the Vietnam War to establish unity in a time of racial tension and discrimination. Dap is an acronym for "dignity and pride" and symbolizes solidarity, a pact taken among soldiers vowing to look after each other. Since then, the fist bump has found a place in popular culture and even in healthcare settings as a more hygienic practice.

A reasonable substitute for the handshake should maintain the essential qualities of a handshake. A new custom should continue to use the upper extremity as many are accustomed to this practice with shaking hands and embracing. It should also allow individuals to face each other to maintain eye contact. When applicable, the gesture may involve brief contact, as human touch is fundamental in communication and vital in human connection, and it conveys kindness and compassion.

We propose a new two-part greeting that establishes rapport without hand, elbow, or foot contact (see photos below). The first part does not require contact and can be performed to acknowledge another at a reasonable distance away—an ideal gesture in a time of social distancing. An individual may simply place their closed fist to their chest just overlying the heart to convey greeting. The second part may be performed only when contact between two parties is permitted. In this scenario, after an individual has placed their fist to their chest, they may extend the forearm outward at a 45 degrees angle. The reciprocating party positions their arm alongside the initiator's arm, and together, they briefly tap their midforearms, forming a cross-like configuration. Important components of the greeting include positioning the palm to face away and making a fist, which directs contaminated fingertips away from others. The cross-like configuration permits the least area of contact, and the brief tap of the forearms minimizes contact time.

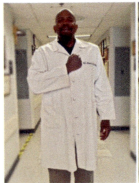 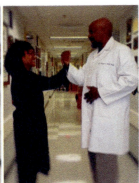 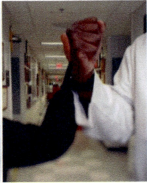

We advocate for adapting to the changing times and altering practice accordingly. This is one idea. The handshake is engrained in many societal practices, and perhaps the changing times have called for a new symbol that conveys strength, maintains solidarity, and ultimately facilitates our healing.[1]

---

1. From Cato T. Laurencin and Aneesah McClinton, The end of the handshake?, https://blogs.sciencemag.org/editors-blog/2020/05/12/the-end-of-the-handshake/. Reprinted with permission from AAAS.

During the COVID period, I took a lesson from Langer and I pushed myself. I pushed my expectations. For that period, I accelerated my career. I was elected to the National Academy of Sciences and the Royal Academy of Engineering (England). I won the Spingarn Medal, the highest award of the NAACP, and won the Hoover Medal, an award given by five engineering societies. I published over 50 papers and patents from our Institute and had 5 grants either funded or renewed. Most of all, I was able to spend time and reconnect with the most important facet of my life, my beautiful and intelligent wife and my beautiful and intelligent children, who mean the most to me.

On my desk, there is a fortune cookie that states, "If you are not happy with what you have, how can you be happy with more?" It is important to always enjoy the moment. It is important as I say to revel in your local happiness. At the same time, it is important to push yourself to new levels and new heights. You must have a certain "impatience with the status quo" while enjoying your "local happiness."

7) Go Beyond Expectations—Theirs and Yours

Somewhere along my own path, I gained the perspective that going beyond expectations was the thing to do. I think it must have started at a fairly young age. I remember telling my parents, "I don't want to be just a doctor." My doctor mother would say, "What do you mean, just a doctor?"

It wasn't until later that I started seeing how science and medicine worked together. Much later I figured out how to pursue both at the same time. I didn't know it back in the conversations with my mother, but looking back, combining the two had always been in the back of my mind.

My parents provided the time, space, and environment where I could think about these things and muddle through what they meant and how I might go after them. They gave me the confidence in my own strengths and abilities, and the conviction that it was alright to take risks to get what I wanted.

We're not all as lucky as I was. Looking back at the Black kids in my first school years, most of them were smarter, more inquisitive, quicker than I was. No question. There are many studies that show that Black children are beyond their peers at ages 3, 4, 5, and 6. But they lose exponentially after first or second grade. What happens is that so many do not have a nurturing environment, and so many get tracked off into side areas.

But in first grade, you aren't yet tracked and pigeonholed. The conditioning hasn't yet sunk in. In first grade, you aren't aware of your limitations; you're still king of the mountain. It's that first-grade mentality that educators have to be able to nourish and tap into, especially those working with Black kids. In this chapter, I talk about how to do that and how to teach kids they need to be "Ray Charles to the bull," in the rapper Lil Wayne's words, that is, to turn a blind eye to stereotyping and stigmatization.

There's an example I use from golfer, Tiger Woods. One of the things Woods was able to do during his peak time was that with all the criticism and marginalization that took place, he was in his way, Ray Charles to the bull. In 2006, after he won the PGA grand slam of golf for the sixth time in 7 years, he was interviewed by sports journalist Jim Huber.

Woods told Huber, "I'm improving, working consistently this year, which is nice, and hopefully I can improve over the winter and be ready for next year." At that time, Woods had gone so far beyond expectations that he seemed almost superhuman.

Huber said, "You're improving? That's a scary thought."

"Well," Woods said, "that's the whole idea."

In my life, I've quietly gone about moving beyond expectations. As a Black person, I've been taught I have to be twice as good to gain half the respect from my peers, and I've found that to be true. Many have thought that would make me angry or discouraged. But I'm not. I speak from a sense of reality.

Black people in America are resilient. Black people in America are loyal to this country. I love America, not only for what the country stands for, but for the hope for what it can become in the future. I think it is important to note that, for all that has been done negatively to Black people in America, we all still embrace democracy, and we all embrace the Republic for which it stands. America is the greatest place to be on earth, and I count myself fortunate to be a part of America. (And I let people know throughout the world when I travel.)

How does one go beyond expectations? First things first. It is important to define yourself and don't let others define you as I described in the first lesson/tip.

Second, it is important to always aim high. Let me give you examples. As an orthopaedic surgeon, it was always important to me that I become the best in my specialty. I worked hard to go to the best medical school (Harvard), the best residency (Harvard), and the best sports medicine and shoulder place (The Hospital for Special Surgery). It's important to hold yourself to being THE BEST. I feel gratified that I have been named to Connecticut's Top Doctors, but more gratified that I have been named to America's Top Doctors for over 15 years.

It is a path that I set long ago. I didn't know it then, but by walking with people smarter than me, I learned that inquiry and being inquiring is the absolute key to advancement in academics. I found that the best clinicians also had labs and were constantly answering questions. I aimed high. I was determined not only to be a great clinician, but to have a big lab, and answer big questions, as a part of my work. These were beyond the expectations of an inner-city kid who was supposed to become an urban family practitioner (which by the way I believe is perhaps the toughest job in America), but I took the job on. I also realized early on that the greatest practitioners, researchers, and clinicians in medicine, engineering, and science were also the greatest teachers and mentors. It is important to not only demonstrate concern and intention, but also to innovate. It is important to create new tools and programs that others can use. I'm proud that we created the first-graduate degree program in regenerative engineering and one of the first NIH-funded graduate PhD programs focusing on Convergence in Regenerative Engineering.

Now, it's all not great news. There are down sides of aiming high. The first and most important is that aiming high and succeed can draw what we call in Philadelphia, the "player-hating" or criticism. This will always be there, and one must get ready for it and used to it. It is the price of success. In my experience, most hate the players and not the game, contrary to popular thought. The second, as I alluded to above is that there can and will be a certain level of marginalization of your achievements. I remember receiving a very prestigious award, one that had never been achieved by anyone in my university, and the university communications person stated, "We'll just place that under our faculty round-up report for the month." I found my prestigious award was listed AFTER an assistant professor's announcement that he reviewed a paper for a journal in dermatology. The late rapper DMX stated it well when he said, "Respect is not expected, but it's given because it's real."

As you continue to aim high and realize your goals, understand that you may not get the level of accolades and response that should occur. But it is important to strive and to aim high for yourself and for others. There are so many young people who are looking for your kind of inspiration. They need to see it so they can believe they too can be it. This is a truth that extends across fields. I receive an email every week, from a high school student who tells me that they have been inspired by me and my work and they are going to a prestigious college. Every month I receive an email or letter from an incarcerated person telling me they are pushing in their studies after reading something that I've written. Awards and recognition are wonderful as acknowledgment of my life's work. But being in the position to inspire young minds and to show them what is possible is why I continue to strive and continue to push on. It's why I am still committed to move beyond the expectations of everyone, and ignore haters and fakes.

Going beyond expectations can be scary. It will test you. The main thing you will encounter is your own personal fear. I relate to you what my father taught me. He was a very no-nonsense man, who spoke in short sentences. He would say "Fear, get over it, life is about taking chances." "Son, Fear, that is someone else's problem." And finally, his most famous saying to me was "Son, failure is not an option." He was serious. And I took it to heart.

Somehow in the love, intimidation, and fearsome respect I had for my father, I absorbed these most important words and incorporated them into my mantra. His comments about fear were important to my upbringing. Martin Luther King said, "We must build dikes of courage to hold back the flood of fear."

While aiming high, my father and both Dr. King acknowledged that fear can occur, and we must combat it head on to succeed. I've done that, and I'm successful because of their collective wisdom.

8) If You're Going to Compete, Make Sure You Have an Unfair Advantage

Once I was giving a lecture at the University of Virginia, talking about how people can advance their careers. "Make sure you have a competitive advantage," I said. Suddenly a shout came from the back of the room. "No! Not a competitive advantage! Make sure you have an unfair advantage!"

The shout came from Anita Jones, the chairperson of UVA's topnotch computer science department. Jones had previously served as director of defense research for the Department of Defense. She had been the head of the Defense Advanced Research Projects Agency (DARPA). She had founded companies. She knew what she was talking about.

Women often tend to be at a competitive disadvantage. Blacks and other minorities are as well. Studies show that if Blacks go into a competitive situation with superior credentials, they do as well as others with equal credentials, but if their credentials are average, they fare badly against others with similarly average credentials. In the Black community, the saying has always been, "If you want to do as well as whites you have to be twice as good." There's still truth to that.

The National Medical Association is the Black counterpart of the AMA. At a talk I gave there for residents and fellows, I asked,"What's your unfair advantage?"

One said, "I graduated from Johns Hopkins Medical School. Now I'm doing my residency at Johns Hopkins."

"Right," I said. "You have a credential that's an advantage for you. It is an advantage that most others will never have. "

My own unfair advantage is that I'm a card-carrying orthopaedic surgeon and a card-carrying engineer. In the right environments, I've got a step-up. The competition is finite; not many have that particular skill set.

The definition of an unfair advantage is very simple:

1. an advantage that you possess;
2. that the other individual or group does not possess;
3. that they will never possess.

You might ask, how do you do this. First you must understand who you are, and what your unique strengths and weaknesses are. The great military strategist Sun Tzu said, "It is crucial to know yourself better than you know your enemy."

Life in many ways is a struggle. As I have stated, it is about triumphs, opportunities, challenges, tests, trials, and hard times. Understanding your strengths is of key importance in your success. Notice that I have removed the word weakness now from the sentence. That is for a reason. My philosophy on strengths states that you should focus 90% of your time on your strengths and 10% of your time addressing your weaknesses. Why? First and foremost, your major advances in life will come because of your strengths. I have interviewed literally thousands of people for jobs, and I have invariably focused on their strengths in making final decisions regarding hiring and promoting people. Second, many times, weaknesses are simply too hard to eliminate. They come with your strengths. For example, your sense of confidence is a great strength, but it may be perceived that you are overconfident. A bit of dilemma, but I for one would hire the confident person. Often weaknesses are part of one's "shadow," the wake behind a fast-moving boat, or the presence behind a great person. Many weaknesses come from being great. That's why I advocate concentrating on strengths.

Your ultimate strength comes from cultivating the unfair advantages. It starts with your taking an inventory of who you are and what you do. What are the things that make you stand out? What are the things in your background and skill set that you have that others don't have and others never will have.

As I stated, it was easy for me. I'm a chemical engineer who is a professor of Chemical Engineering and was named as one of the 100 Engineers of the Modern Era by the American Institute of Chemical Engineers and at the same time, and I'm a board-certified orthopaedic surgeon with extra expertise in the area of shoulder and knee surgeon. So my work takes advantages of this "unfair advantage" in the work I do as a scientist and a surgeon.

Second, follow the advice of Peter F. Drucker, management consultant, educator, and author, who emphasized that it was important to know your strengths, know how you perform, and know your values. It is really a combination of these factors that determine your success in life. Especially in the workplace, your personal understanding of how you perform and what is important to you value wise will make huge difference in the success of your life.

Third, look to people in your profession who are already cultivating their unfair advantage. How are they doing it, and what lessons can you glean from their journey.

9) If You Do Good Things, Good Things Happen

This is one of the rules I try hard to instill in my working groups and in those I mentor.

At my Institute, I've told my staff that any decisions we make have to

1. be the right thing to do;
2. be the legal thing to do;
3. have optics that are confirm the decisions are right and legal; and
4. be a good thing to do.

I know there can be a number of definitions, when using the term "good,". For this lesson, I define the first "good" in the statement as being analogous to "possessing or displaying moral virtue." The second "good" is analogous to "something of benefit or advantage." So, translating this, carrying out something that displays high moral virtue or value, will bring about great benefits to you. Doing the right thing and doing the legal thing are nice and are important. Doing the virtuous thing is at the next level. It can sometimes be hard, especially if there are competing interest around you.

When I served as Vice President for Health Affairs at the University of Connecticut, there was a well-known program for some faculty. They would have their salary increase by enormous amounts for 1 year, and then they would retire the next year. Since their retirement salary was based on their highest income, they would receive an enormous boost in their retirement income. If that weren't enough, the faculty were then rehired by the University at 40%—50% time. The amount determined was just enough to keep their high overall salaries when they retired by a combination of retirement income and continued part-time salary by the University. Overnight, these individuals went from highly paid people working 100% time, to equally highly paid people working on 40% time in some cases.

When I started as Vice President, I examined the program and thought it was unfair to the taxpayers of the state. I also thought it was unfair to the young faculty members as often the rehired retiree faculty were not active and utilized resources that could go to the younger, more active faculty. I decided to put an end to the program. It was the right thing to do, it was the legal thing to do (for those not under contract or whose contracts were up for renewal), and most of all, it was a good thing to do.

It was an unpopular decision. Many senior faculty had become so accustomed to the rehired retiree program that they thought that "the deal" as it was called was their right. But it was a good decision in that it was morally virtuous.

A few months after I ended the program, I received a call from representatives of the Connecticut state legislature and the Governor's office. They were disturbed in hearing about a special "deal" for faculty where they would continue to be paid 100% of their salary by the state and at the same time only work for 40% time. They wanted to meet with me as the head of the medical center. This was one of my first meetings with the state legislature and the Governor office. The first question cut to the quick. Did the program they describe exist? This was followed with a statement that if it did there would be negative consequences both for the medical center and for me. I answered clearly and succinctly. When I arrived at the medical center, the program existed and actually faculty had every expectation to continue joining on. I ended the program months before.

My statement brought knowing nods from State Representatives, Senators, and a nod from the Governor's office representative. To this day, I believe this meeting was responsible for the excellent relationship I've continued to have with the legislature of the State of Connecticut. I did the right thing, the virtuous thing. In the end good things happened, such as a relationship of trust with the legislature and Governor's office, savings to the medical center as we achieved the first balanced budget in years there, and improved resources for younger faculty to carry out their research, teaching, and clinical work. If you do good things, good things happen.

When I first started at Harvard Medical School, I actually was enrolled in the MD–MPP program. I admired the senior professors who had taken on administration and policy roles. I particularly admired President William Bowen, the President of Princeton when I was there. As a member of the University Council Executive Committee, I frequently had the opportunity to interact with him. He was smart, kind, humble, and magnanimous. Inside, he had the heart of a lion. He was a scholar and humanitarian. He was an early champion of Blacks at Princeton. The substantial numbers of Blacks arrived during his tenure as President. Perhaps most notably he cowrote the book, "The Shape of the River: Long-Term Consequences of Considering Race in College and University Admissions." The book was a landmark tome on affirmative action. Detailing the most comprehensive study on the subject, President Bowen provided evidence on how race-sensitive admissions policy actually work for the benefit of all.

The world had the opportunity to know him as I did, a lion. In May of 2014, he was invited to Haverford College to be the commencement speaker. He was actually the substitute commencement speaker. Robert Birgeneau, the former chancellor of the University of California at Berkeley, was to speak (and get an honorary degree)

William Bowen, former president of Princeton University, used his commencement speech at Haverford College outside Philadelphia to criticize students who campaigned against Robert Birgeneau, former chancellor of the University of California, Berkeley. A group at Haverford protested Birgeneau's coming to speak. Instead, the group provided a long list of demands including the writing of a letter to Haverford students on "what you have learned from them." The protests stemmed from his handling of an event in 2011 where police engaged students who were protesting.

At commencement, President Bowen stated: "I am disappointed that those who wanted to criticize Birgeneau's handling of events at Berkeley chose to send him such an intemperate list of 'demands.'"

"In my view," he said, "they should have encouraged him to come and engage in a genuine discussion, not to come, tail between his legs, to respond to an indictment that a self-chosen jury had reached without hearing counter-arguments."

Bowen also said Birgeneau had "responded intemperately, failing to make proper allowance for the immature, and, yes, arrogant inclinations of some protesters. Aggravated as he had every right to be, I think he should be with us today." He then said Birgeneau had "responded intemperately, failing to make proper allowance for the immature, and, yes, arrogant inclinations of some protesters. Aggravated as he had every right to be, I think he should be with us today."

As I have taught earlier, always walk with someone smarter than you. I did that with President Bowen.

But, back to the story. I arrived at Harvard Medical School, and two things happened. First, I realized that a large number of people who work in policy areas are actually not policy people. They don't have Master's in Public Policy, they are great people in their own world, and they are selected for policy positions. I realized that was the case for President Bowen. At the same time, I had a growing desire to return to my engineering roots, which led me to MIT, which led me to Professor Robert Langer, and which led me to make a critical decision whether or not to pursue and MD–PhD program.

Believe it or not, many people tried to discourage me from undertaking a combined MD and PhD program. Initially the MD–PhD program admitted me, but did not provide funding to me. That made it almost impossible to pursue. In the midst of this, a senior Dean at Harvard Medical School called me to his office. He had a solution for me. "What if we were to pay for your entire medical school education, including a stipend?" I was in disbelief. He repeated his offer with some emphasis now, "What if we were to pay for your ENTIRE medical school education including stipend?"

"You would of course not be pursing the MD–PhD." I was a bit flabbergasted on a couple of levels. As this was Harvard Medical School, my expectation was that I would receive nothing but encouragement for pursuing an academic program, instead I was being discouraged. Second, I was sitting in the room with a senior Dean with no funding offered by the institution to pursue my MD–PhD, but funding for the rest of my MD, if I would forget pursuing an MD–PhD. I had to make a decision. Do I pursue the MD–PhD, and possibly have a zillion dollars of debt, or complete my MD, with my hefty tuition, fees, and stipend paid for by the school. As you may surmise (since you have read my biography by this point in the book), I decided on the MD–PhD. The overall reason was based on considering what was the "good" thing to do. Yes, doing the right thing was important, but doing the good thing was the overwhelming factor. Asking myself what the virtuous thing to do, a number of answers came through. My parents were strong believers in education "Get all that you can," they would say to me. Getting two doctorates definitely checked that box. Also, making a grand contribution to society and perhaps changing the world, yes, I liked that possibility. I saw it happening more with a combined degree. And finally, I just didn't like the fact that I was denied funding for my combined program, and given funding for the single program. It seemed unvirtuous.

So yes, I pursued the combined program. I often say that after meeting and marrying my wife, it is the best and most gratifying decision I ever made. Truly good things (beneficial things) have happened as a result. If you do good things, good things happen.

10) You Know What You Know, but You Don't Know What You Don't Know

During my first year as Vice President for Health Affairs and Dean and head of the health center at the University of Connecticut, the senior leadership team and I had a discussion. Our internal medicine group was losing millions of dollars a year. Typically, internal medicine/primary care in an integrated medical center can lose between $60,000 and $80,000 per year, per doctor. One just cannot pay enough to primary doctors because of all the ancillary people they depend on and utilize. The question was: What should we do?

Given the losses, the senior strongly recommended disbanding the primary care group. UConn Health would be out of the primary care medicine business and have all specialists. The numbers were checked and rechecked I was told. A growing bandwagon started to build to proceed. There was a lot pressure for me to do this as the "group" was together on this, and I inherited a large deficit at UConn Health on arrival.

The argument to close the group seemed persuasive enough. But before I agreed to move forward, I drew from the lesson, "You know what you know, but you don't know what you don't know." I asked a very simple question. If we disband the group, you've shown me what we will save, but what will use. Evidently the team putting together numbers had the savings in income of doctors, office space, staff figured down to the penny, but did not know the numbers on downside of not having a primary care group. "Do we know what our losses will be in terms of referrals these doctors will be making to other systems since they don't work for us. What about ancillary income from testing (such as lab tests and X-rays). How much income do they generate from say MRI referrals?

When we studied that, we found that the primary care group brought in 10 times the amount they cost us. If their loss was two million, their gain to the hospital was 20 million. When this was brought out at the senior team meeting, some were speechless, and others denied having supported the closure of the group. A couple repeated my lesson phrase "You know what you know, but you don't know what you don't know." I said "good" to them. It meant we were making progress.

Whenever information is brought to bear about a position we should take, I've learned to explore the negatives as thoroughly as I can. Often (as happened in our primary group problem) people may be very quick to decide without knowing what the unknowns are. And if something seems clear enough, there's commonly a mutual reinforcement or bandwagon effect that can influence you, as a leader, as well.

If someone's advocating something, I need to hear what the contrary view is. I want to understand that, and I want to get as much of a grip as possible on what it is that we don't know. That why minority reports—reports that have a plan contrary to the group hold weight with me. They are often have embedded "You know what you know, but you don't know what you don't know" information.

Now the truth is that many decisions have to be made in life, especially in medicine and academics and engineering, where one does not have the luxury of a lot of time in making decisions.

Colin Powell has a view of this in terms of leadership. He argues that there's a spectrum of information that allows you to make a decision—he talks about a 40%–70% range. Under 40%, you don't have as much information as you need to make the decision. Over 70% of the case may be relatively clear. But somewhere in that zone—P40 to P70—you have enough to move forward. If you don't act, you may lose the opportunity.

How do I think about making decisions? First, I try to tap into my intuitive sense. What does my intuition tell me? When I use the term intuition, I don't mean the hair on the back of my neck. I think of it as the sum total of all of the information gathering that I have done in life, applied to this particular decision or problem. Psychologist Gary Klein, an expert in what he calls naturalistic decision-making, has stated that 90% of the important decisions we make are based on intuition. Intuition can be managed and grown as a learnable art, a part of your emotional quotient skill set. If your intuitive sense is supported by the information gathered, then proceed with your decision.

The value of your intuitive sense has been known for centuries. For example:

> *I learned that when it eases your mind to do a thing, it's right; and when it don't ease your mind, you better go slow.*
>
> Henry Martin, bell-ringer, University of Virginia, 1914.

Intuition is key. What do you do if the information gathered doesn't support the conclusions you've come to? The first thing to do is to ask the question, do the people brining the information know more about this than I do? Next there needs to be a reevaluation of the information, especially the sources to determine if the information is valid. If your intuitive sense is not supported by the information gathered, then ask the question, do the people bringing the info to me know more about this than I do? If you are more knowledgeable than the people bringing the info, or the information is not valid, follow your intuitive sense.

If the information is valid, and the people around you are more knowledgeable than you, that is the case you lean toward following more of the informational path over the intuitive path. Construct a plan that makes sure that at each step, the consequences are measured as changes are made. Finally execute the plan, with close follow-up.

Decision-making can make people unhappy. Not all decisions create universal happiness. There is the amusing story of two boys fighting over a ball, and the wise minister saw them. He stopped them and asked why they were fighting. The first boy gave the reasons why the ball was his. After a moment, the minister decided, "YOU ARE RIGHT." The second boy then responded and gave the reasons why the ball was his. The minister after a moment then decided "YOU ARE RIGHT." The parents of the children saw what occurred and ran over to the minister, and both said, how can you tell each of our sons hat they were right? After a moment, the minister made the decision, "YOU ARE BOTH RIGHT!"

Decision-making, especially in complex organizations, can be a tight-rope. As Dr. Martin Luther King, Jr. said "All progress is precarious, and the solution of one problem brings us face to face with another problem." Successful people make many decisions, and some (hopefully most) go well and some do not. As I described earlier in the book, it is important to learn from things that happen whether they be good or bad. One way we can categorize them are miscues, mistakes, and blunders.

11) When Decisions Go Wrong

Miscues: Things you attempted to do, and they were the right thing to do, but you did not accomplish things or it didn't work out. This is the Laurencin 15% −30% Rule of life. There should be a certain percentage of time that you will attempt to do something, especially something big and will not succeed. This is not necessarily a bad thing since it means you are striving.

Mistakes could be defined as the things you attempted to do, and you thought they were the right things to do, but it turned not to be the right thing to do, and you did not accomplish t or it didn't work out. Again, this is not necessarily a terrible thing. There is a learning process that takes places with mistakes being made and processing these in your intuition armamentarium.

There is an African proverb that states "Do not look where you fell, but where you slipped"— analyzing your mistakes can be one of the hardest things you do. It's humbling, but it also provides growth opportunities. For example, every day in hospitals across the country, incident reports of breaches in the quality of patient care are handled by quality care people and a committee of individuals that report to or are a part of the board of directors. Their job is to seek to analyze problems that come up so that they do not come up again. Outstanding hospitals embrace the process and are firmly on the runway toward excellence in care.

Blunders: Things you attempted to do, from the start these things or decisions were not the right thing to do, you sensed or knew it from the start, and you did not accomplish things or it didn't work out. A goal in life is to minimize and/or avoid the blunders. The fact is you gain little from blunders because you already knew the decisions were not right from the start.

Remember to use your intuition. It is a valuable tool. Always remember, You Know What You Know, But You Don't Know What You Don't Know.

12) Reasonable People Act Reasonably (and Unreasonable People Don't)

I probably use this rule a zillion times every day. I use it when forming collaborations with people, when undertaking new research projects, and when deciding how far I can rely on others' judgments. I love working with people who are reasonable. I love working with good people. I seek them out when collaborating on projects, I seek them out when forming friendships. Life is too short to bring unreasonable people in your life. Most times you have a choice.

Relationships begin the moment that you meet someone. There is a lot of reliance on your intuitive sense as I discussed in the last lesson. There's also a lot of reliance on your own emotional quotient in judging what the person stands for, and whether you will get along. The beginnings are important. It's where you get your best gage of what the person is like. You have an opportunity to understand how the relationship might play out in the future. (Another of my rules of thumb comes into play here: "If the courtship is rough, the marriage is likely to be rougher."). As an engineer and scientist, this is particularly true. The early interactions allow you to judge the level of advice or proposals or arguments an individual will bring to the table later on.

A case in point is a situation that happened when I was chair of the Department of Orthopaedic Surgery at the University of Virginia. We were recruiting a brilliant surgeon from another institution. During the recruitment period, we liked everything we saw. We wanted him.

At the other institution, he was a senior associate professor. But our evaluators felt he wasn't qualified to be a full professor yet, close, but he would have to come in as an associate with tenure. Then after a year or two, he could probably move up to full professor Additionally, I wanted to provide him with an endowed chair. But it's unusual for associate professors to be given endowed chairs. We'd have to apply for that. There were no guarantees, but I would do my best to make it happen.

He wasn't happy about all of this. He was counting on coming in as a full professor, and an endowed chair was a big incentive for him to switch institutions. I had reasonable assurances about the endowed chair, and I thought we wouldn't have any problems elevating his rank later on. But there were no guarantees, and moving sideways from one institution to another, or even a little backward, wasn't going to do good things for either his career or his reputation.

We discussed these things back and forth. I really got to know him, and he got to know me. In the end, it came down to my saying to him—Listen, we've gotten to know each other. You know me, I know you. You have to have a certain level of trust that this will work out. I hope you can bring yourself to trust me on it.

He called back and said, Okay, I do trust you. If I come here, you're the chairman and in many ways, I'm already putting my career in your hands. So, yes, I'll proceed.

I judged him from those interactions to be a reasonable person. He acted reasonably. He had a serious problem to solve and he was careful, thoughtful, and analytical in how he went about it. I knew that if an issue came up in the future, those were qualities he would bring to bear on it.

He came to the University of Virginia and received an associate professor appointment with tenure. His nomination to receive a prestigious endow chair in the department was approved. Two years later, he went up for full professor, and it was approved.

This professor turned out to be one of the most reasonable faculty members in the department. He was an "ambassador of Quan" in many ways for me. He can explain my philosophy, how I can be trusted and am devoted to the welfare of my faculty. I valued his support, but above all I valued his friendship.

On the other hand, I've had opportunities for partnerships and collaborations in which the preliminaries haven't seemed right and I've said "pass," even knowing that the association might be successful. I remember times in which people tried to persuade me to work with people, who I felt were not honest or reasonable. This was early in my career, and the people we were talking about were career influencers. I am proud that I stuck to my principles and did the good/virtuous thing. Good things happened after that.

I've had the opposite experiences as well, situations where I had preliminary doubts about a person's ability to be reasonable but I was persuaded by other factors into going in with them anyway. These times have been very few and very far between. For the most part, my initial impressions have been right. I've learned from the experiences, and it's helped me build my intuitive senses.

That's what makes Reasonable People Act Reasonably (and unreasonable people don't), such an important lesson to understand and follow.

Today I'm governed by the important principle of the great Maya Angelou. She taught, "When people show you who they are, believe them." Most of my decisions regarding my associations are based upon the honesty and reasonableness of people. Sometimes people show their true colors over time. While I am reluctant to cut ties in relationships with colleagues and even friends, Maya Angelou's words have had more importance to me over time. Relationships evolve, and as you learn about people, unreasonableness may be seen. Remembering that unreasonable people will not act reasonably is important and managing relationships those that are great and not so great.

Leaders need to build groups and associations. They need to tie people to them, and more often than not they have to make relatively quick judgments. But the "reasonable" principle holds good whether you're a leader or not, whenever you are contemplating a close interaction with someone.

13) The Three Things You Should be Able to Say: "I Don't Know"; "I'm Sorry"; "I Love You"

In the Massachusetts General Hospital's Orthopaedic Surgery Residency, we used to have morning rounds with Dr. Henry Mankin, the King of Boston's Orthopaedic Surgery mecca, a man of towering stature. These were called "breakfast rounds," which was a misnomer since Dr. Mankin was the only one who ate. The rest of us were so scared we might be called on that we kept a low profile. Every once in a while, a new intern or resident would come in with a bowl of corn flakes. That person would be called on all week, and the lessons were sometimes meted out brutally. This was more than 30 years ago. Teaching young doctors has now been transformed, and such practices have been abandoned. But in the 1980s and 1990s, this was the norm.

Despite his occasional harshness, Dr. Mankin cared deeply for his trainees, which we all knew. He taught us orthopaedic surgery, but he also taught us lessons for life. He was deeply invested in all of us. This was not only during our residency training but throughout our lives. Just after my son was born years after I completed residency, I received a very touching letter from Dr. Mankin directed to my son. It offered him admission to the Harvard Orthopaedic Surgery residency program, the spot to begin in 2022.

Dr. Mankin also taught us of the art of Hattage, which has been so eloquently written on in the literature. The principal of Hattage states there are times that doing less for a patient is more. Don't be afraid to take a step back and ask what is truly helpful for a patient, instead of throwing technology or surgery at a problem.

Dr. Mankin insisted that there were three things you had to be able to say to be a successful human being, a "mensch," in his words: "I don't know," "I'm sorry," and "I love you." He explained why these three things are important and how they grow in importance as you progress through the different phases of life.

All three can be difficult to say. For doctors especially, "I don't know" can be hard. And among doctors, maybe for Mass General/Harvard trained doctors most of all. You have to feel very comfortable with yourself to admit such a thing. "I'm sorry" is almost unheard of in a clinical situation, but sometimes it is truly called for, and whether you're able to muster the courage to say it can be a sure measure of your humanity.

"I love you" is little bit different. But that depth of appreciation is hardly ever articulated among attending physicians and their trainees. Once after Dr. Mankin had reiterated his three phrase mantra again, we were looking at a difficult case during breakfast rounds.

"How would you diagnose this?" Dr. Mankin asked the chief resident.

"I don't know, Dr. Mankin" the chief resident said.

"Good," said Mankin. "You have to be able to say that."

"How about you?" he asked a second resident.

"I don't know," said the second.

"Good," said Mankin.

On it went. "I don't know." "Good." "I don't know." "Good." "I don't know." "Good." Until it was my turn.

"And what do you think this is, Dr. Laurencin?" he asked.

"I love you, Dr. Mankin, I said.

There was a hush in the room. I had dared to say this to Dr. Mankin. The lull continued for a few seconds, until Dr. Mankin burst into laughter. This signaled the timid resident crew in the room (over 20) to proceed with smiles and laughter too.

But that breakfast rounds affected me forever. There are actually four things we have trouble saying as people. "I don't know, I'm sorry, I was wrong, and I love you." Because of the breakfast rounds, I am quicker to express those feelings quicker to acknowledge each of these feelings, and quick to let people know around me, that it is ok for them to express these feelings.

I don't know.

"The fool doth think he is wise, but the wise man knows himself to be a fool." This is what Shakespeare wrote. Stating that you don't know, especially in a group of leaders, can be transformative. It can make people think out of the box and make people question the core of what they believe. For me, it was exhilarating at Harvard Medical School to have a senior professor in immunology tell me that he did not know the answer, but invited me to speculate. Great professors in orthopaedic surgery said the same thing to me. That's perhaps why I am an orthopaedic surgery. There is a certain amount of honesty and authenticity that comes with the statement, I don't know.

I'm sorry.

I apologize a lot. The alarm goes off in the morning and it wakes my wife. I leave my driveway, and a car comes down the street … maybe I was coming down the driveway to fast? I review the work for the day, and there are a few things that are slipping through the cracks with my team. There are no bad team members, just leaders who could be doing their job better, so I apologize. Saying I'm sorry and/or apologizing is important in life. It speaks of empathy and sensitivity, and it emphasizes that in the end we are all in it together. It is one of my favorite phases.

I was wrong.

For most people, it is very hard to admit being wrong. We are just programmed to be right. Actually, we are programmed to be righteous. We are programmed to believe that what we are doing is just and proper, and so of course it must be right. Wrong is a strong opposite of right, and it's a place that people have a hard time going to.

But we all should. Self-critique is important. Well, maybe not to the point that you become depressed, but introspection can be helpful. And when that critique demonstrates one was wrong, be ready to admit it. And next work to remedy the issue or problem.

I love you.

These are three words that can never be said enough. Never lose an opportunity to say this to loved ones. It is an expression that is never worn out or hackneyed. It also reinforces why we are in this business called life.

14) Better Together Than Best Apart

These words come from Dr. Mohammed Attawia. I first met him at MIT when I opened my lab there. I was a 20 something youngster fresh from my PhD. I had worked hard to get grant funding. I really had to, or they were going to close my lab. In the first year, I had two grants from the National Institutes of

Health and one grant from the National Science Foundation. I was flying. But I needed help. I was advised not to obtain postdoctoral fellows, to invest in graduate students instead, and master's students in particular. That advice didn't seem especially smart, and the source, the Dean of Science's office, didn't appear to be in my best interest. So, I ignored it, and I hired two postdoctoral fellows under my grants. One was Mohammed Attawia.

Mohammed had a wealth of talents. He was born in Egypt and was trained in medicine, as a pediatrician. He had extra training in research that made him a great addition for someone working in biomedical research. Although he wasn't an engineer, he took to the work and the projects quickly. He really was supersmart. At the same time, he was a bit of a philosopher. He was able to distill issues and problems with his philosophy that could be explained in one short line.

His most important philosophy to me was "Better Together than Best Apart."

This mantra says that in making decisions and moving forward in medicine, business, and life, it's better to make the decision that everyone can agree on rather than the one a single person might think is the best, even when that person is the leader. It also means that the best decision is inherently not the best decision if it cannot be accepted by the group.

One of the key areas where this is true is in the operating room. When I'm operating along with my senior residents, I make sure that we're in agreement. Even though I'm the professor, it's a collaboration. If we're doing a difficult shoulder or knee surgical operation, the pathway that we all agree on is the pathway we normally take.

In the field of surgery, we have transitioned considerably from a world where there was one leader and one opinion. When we're in the operating room, we do what we call a "hard timeout." Everybody stops. We identify the patient, the procedure. And every single person in that room has to agree that it's okay to proceed. Years ago, it was unheard that the scrub nurse would tell the surgeon whether or not it's okay to proceed. But now that's standard procedure. If your goals are excellence, reliability, and consistency of outcomes, that is what you do. It's Better Together than Best Apart.

My staff are often surprised when I ask them what they think we should do. Sometimes the reply is, "well you're the boss." But it shouldn't be. Answers should bubble up from the group. Dr. Martin Luther King, Jr. stated. A genuine leader is not a searcher for consensus but a molder of consensus. I like to work with teams to come up with answers. My role is not to create the answers but to mold consensus of the group to bring answers together.

One thing that I always do, with the teams that I lead is to place time in the schedule for a roundtable of talks. Often individuals have intended an entire meeting and have great ideas, but no opportunities to have them heard. I learned this from my colleague and friend Norman Augustine, the former Chairman and President of Lockheed. Individuals around the table are gratified with being able to express their thoughts during a roundtable. It helps to preserve the concept of better together than best apart.

If you're a fan of Start Trek, you might think of the progression seen in the Star Trek series. In the prequel, Enterprise, the captain was on deck barking orders. He often actually decided on plans and courses of action contrary to his crew. Next came Captain James T. Kirk. He sat in the center with his people arrayed around him. He asked questions now and then and listened. But then he made the decision. In the last iteration, Star Trek Next Generation, Captain Jean Luc Picard, had two others sitting with him on the deck. He relied on his team when it came to decision time. At his left actually sat a ship's counselor, denoting the importance and value of working as a team. It was rare to see Captain Picard take a course of action without some level of consensus.

That's the way the world moved during the years the Star Trek series were developed. Knowing it not, the world has adopted the lesson "Better Together than Best Apart." Many industries have taken up that same mentality, most famously the airline industry. The great, and tragic, game changing event there was the world's worst airline catastrophe, when 500 people died in a collision of a Pan Am plane and a KLM plane on the runway in Amsterdam. The Dutch pilot, KLM's senior instructor, had looked at the situation and said, "We're going." On the recording, you can hear the copilot's nervousness, but he was afraid to contradict the pilot. Nowadays, there has to be a consensus before they move forward.

In businesses and other organizations, the leader needs to take into account the opinion of others. Not only because that's usually the way to reach a good outcome, but because it brings people together. It lets others know they're important; it tells them they are part of a team. To have people rally around, to support making the final idea happen, they need to feel that they are part of it, that they have skin in the game.

Of course, if you, the leader, believe there is one much better way and the other ways aren't workable, you have to make a command decision. In that case, staff working with you are more likely to support you if they know you are reasonable, that you've compromised in the past, and that you are a collaborative person who takes their views seriously. That allows you to get buy-in. And you have to have put money into the buy-in meter, because there is no question that down the line you are going to need it.

Underlying all of this is a simple concept—everyone important and everyone's input matter. At one University of Virginia commencement, the speaker, a famous professor, said to the students—"You keep us young, you keep us on our toes. Your insight helps us to be better. Your knowledge challenges us."

Better Together than Best Apart.

15) Celebrate Your Successes 10 Times More Than Any Setbacks

As I stated earlier, life is about triumphs, opportunities, challenges, trials, and hardships. We grow from them all.

Everyone knows how to benefit from triumphs and opportunities. But what of challenges. The truth is that we must take on challenges as opportunities. Most of my major academic achievements have come by way of obstacles placed in my way. Whether it be the closure of my department, or the initial underfunding of my research program, these challenges represent real opportunities. I've been called a survivor. Many ask, "how does he do it?" I have embraced a philosophy learned from others, and I teach it.

First understand that "Tough Times Go Away, Tough People Don't." Also understand that "The Toughest Times often don't get tougher, but tough people do." Louisa May Alcott once said, "I am not afraid of storms, for I am learning how to sail my ship." In dealing with trials and hardships, Albert Camus once said "In the depth of winter, I finally learned that within me there lay an invincible summer."

Second, trust yourself, know yourself, and believe in yourself. Earlier in the book I spoke of the work of Sun Tzu and the importance of knowing yourself. But his philosophy is beyond that. You must not only know yourself, but you also have to believe in yourself. Third, we are defined by how we "Stand the Rain." This is one of my favorite songs written by Jimmy Jam and Terry Lewis and sung by one of my favorite groups, New Edition. They grew up in the Roxbury neighborhood of Boston, Massachusetts, and formed their group in 1978. They grew up in the same inner-city environment that I did and are in many ways kindred spirits. Their song speaks to the full panoply of triumphs, opportunities, challenges, trials, and hardships that take place in life. It speaks to all the storms that life throws at you as you go through the challenges on the path to success. Some professionally successful people—no matter what field—will create a narrative of their journey to make it all look easy. They might leave you thinking that all the pieces fell together easily at every step of the path. But I can tell you that if you peek behind the curtain, you will see all the obstacles, mistakes, and challenges—all the storms it took to get to where they are. And if you've lived long enough you know that this is the stuff of life. There is always something. How you get through it is most often based on how you gird up to stand the storms and rain. While this inspires me across my entire life, I can say absolutely that I have been blessed with a wife and partner who has been through the storms with me, and I with her. Not only have we built a family and a life, but she has given me unconditional love, guidance, and support. It's like building a rock-solid foundation that you can trust and count on. We all go through storms, but if you have someone by your side to whom you are committed, and they are committed to you, it sure makes it easier. I recommend to everyone to find a life partner to help you "Stand the Rain." I often quote a University of Tokyo study where rodents were first shocked with electricity and levels of stress hormones were measured. The levels were high. Next rodents were shocked again, but in some of the cages, a companion rodent was placed before. The rodents with companions had lower levels of stress hormones when they were shocked than those without. Having a companion will not keep you from avoiding the rain, but they will help to see you through the rain.

My philosophy of life has been to embrace the challenges, and even trials and hardships as opportunities for success and even greatness. The bible teaches us:

This small and temporary trouble we suffer will bring us tremendous and eternal joy, much greater than the trouble. For we fix our attention, not on things that are seen, but on things that are unseen. What can be seen lasts only for a time, but what cannot be seen lasts forever.

2 Corinthians 4. 17−18

The bible also teaches us that:

For which cause we FAINT NOT.

But that though our outward man may perish, our inward man is renewed day by day.

2 Corinthians 4. 16 (King James)

I believe that our greatness lies in tackling problems and achieving through adversities. We know that if there is no struggle, there is no progress. We also know that power yields nothing without a struggle, it never did, and it never will. There principles have been taught to us by Frederick Douglas. When struggles occur, attitude is everything. General Patton said, "Always advance. Never dig in." And, as I constantly teach, it is important to remember the Zimbabwe proverb, that "To stumble is not to fall but go faster."

Taking on the full range of life, especially trials and hardships is important for success. Dr. Martin Luther King said, "the ultimate measure of a man is not where he stands in moments of comfort and convenience, but where he stands at times of challenge and controversy." Those few powerful words define a mindset bent on success.

I learned a lot about mindset from Dr. Leon Eisenberg. Eisenberg was a phenomenon. The chairman of psychiatry first at Johns Hopkins then at Harvard, he was, as one colleague described him, "the pivotal person in 20th century child psychiatry." He more or less single handedly built the field of social medicine, pioneering mental health research in poor countries, studying disparities in healthcare, and initiating programs that combined medicine and the humanities, or more precisely, humanitarianism. Not incidentally, he was instrumental in bringing diversity to Harvard Medical School, pushing to significantly expand the negligible number of Black students and maintaining Harvard's commitment as chairman of the admissions committee.

This man, another of the giants of modern medicine, had had his own share of troubles. From Philadelphia, he had been denied admission to the University of Pennsylvania Medical School, which in his day severely restricted the number of Jews. After a state legislator intervened, he enrolled and 4 years later graduated first in his class. Despite this, his application for an internship at the University of Pennsylvania Hospital was rejected, along with those of the seven other Jewish applicants.

Other trials awaited Eisenberg in his life, none that I knew about them when I was a student and resident. When I began my career, Eisenberg kept in touch, always with words of advice and encouragement. I understood as the years went by that he and his wife, Carola (the medical school's dean of student affairs), were still monitoring my progress. I'm sure they were doing the same for many of the others they helped along the way.

In 2007, I heard that Eisenberg was ill with prostate cancer. One day, I received a note from him. He was in hospice, he said. He felt he was in his last days and he wanted to send a message. This, his last message, was that he had lived a good life, but he also reflected on how many people had tried to keep him down. Now, at the end of his days, he felt he had focused too much on the negatives. If he could do it over again, he said, he would have celebrated his triumphs much more than dwelling on his setbacks. That was his message to me. We should make sure to celebrate our triumphs.

In honor of Dr. Leon Eisenberg, I tell everyone to celebrate your triumphs 10 times more than any setbacks. Realize and celebrate the blessing that you can. Life is too short to spend dwelling on the "shoulda, couldas." Celebrate the "been there and done that," often—at least 10 times more. I think that's what Dr. Eisenberg would want us to do.

16) Success Is Not What You've Done. It's What You Leave Behind

In late 2007, Harvard's Judah Folkman visited my lab at the University of Virginia. Two months later, he was dead of a heart attack that hit him as he ran to catch a plane in the Denver airport. The photograph I have of him in my Virginia lab is one of my most treasured possessions.

Dr. Folkman was one of the very greatest medical scientists of modern times. He was the smartest man at Harvard. I told the story on this early in the book. I cannot begin to even estimate how much I learned from him both when I was a student and afterward. But I think I learned as much from him in his death as I did in his life.

Dr. Folkman's life was a full one; he had a wonderful family, students who admired and respected him, great colleagues, and friends. As in all great men, his success came with struggle. Many of his theories were not immediately embraced as happens with most trailblazers. But by the end of his career, he was recognized as the person he was. He was a fabulous clinician and a world-renowned scientist.

I was invited to come to his memorial service after he died. The service was in Boston. At his memorial service, people came from around the country and around the world. Folkman had combined extraordinary brilliance with a deeply compassionate nature that made him beloved by his patients, students, and colleagues. The gathering at his memorial included luminaries from the world of medicine, patients he had healed, physicians he had trained, a large cohort of friends, and, of course, family.

It seemed to me as I watched it seemed almost as if the mourners could be divided into three distinct groups. The first group were the people he had mentored. They talked about how he had taught and guided them, what his example had meant to them, and how he had changed their lives through the example of his life. The second group were those who spoke about his quest to make a difference to the world, his creation of the anticancer drug Avastin, the naysayers he had, the career struggles he had to overcome. The third group was the most important group. They were his family. They knew him the most. They knew him as the loving, generous person that he was. They cried for him.

Reflecting on that memorial service, it seemed to me that the three groups conveyed a profound lesson. I also experienced a moment. I realized that Dr. Folkman had even taught me in death as he had taught me so much in life. Success in life is really what you leave behind. One group are the students, the colleagues, and the circle of people who he worked with and interacted with. They like me, continue to say his name, and spread the work on the great things he stood for and embodied. Dr. Folkman touched these people, individually through his friendship, teaching, mentoring, and through the great example he set. So, one area defining your success are the students and colleagues that you have. The second area of emphasis is the contribution he made to society. His theories and work lead to new drug treatments that resulted in (and continue to) the savings of perhaps millions of people's lives.

In Judah Folkman's case, his contributions were absolutely prodigious, but really everyone is capable of leaving this world a better place in some way, answering Martin Luther King's "most urgent question": What have you done for others? So, the second area defining your success is your contributions to humanity. How are you helping the human condition? That should be a question you pose and strive to answer on a daily basis. The third group is your family: the people who know you the most, who love you the most, and who care for you the most. So, the third area defining your success is family. From the memorial service, Dr. Folkman taught me that family was the most important thing. Those who care for you most deeply are your family, your immediate circle of loved ones. They are the most important thing in your life, not your business, your work, or your career, however, satisfying or even exhilarating those might be. Remember that.

So, I have given you some insight into how I got here and some of the lessons I have learned along the way, but I also want I want to share my resume as another insight into my journey.

Cato T. Laurencin, MD, PhD, is the University Professor and Albert and Wilda Van Dusen Distinguished Endowed Professor of Orthopaedic Surgery at the University of Connecticut. He is a professor of Chemical Engineering, a professor of Materials Science and Engineering, and a professor of Biomedical Engineering at the school. He serves as the chief executive officer of the Connecticut Convergence Institute for Translation in Regenerative Engineering and the director of the Raymond and Beverly Sackler Center for Biomedical, Biological, Physical and Engineering Sciences at UConn.

Dr. Laurencin earned a BSE in Chemical Engineering from Princeton University, and his MD, Magna Cum Laude, from the Harvard Medical School, and received the Robinson Award for Surgery. He earned his PhD in Biochemical Engineering/Biotechnology from the Massachusetts Institute of Technology where he was named a Hugh Hampton Young Fellow. A practicing sports medicine and shoulder surgeon, Dr. Laurencin has been named to America's Top Doctors for over 15 years. He is a fellow of the American Academy of Orthopaedic Surgeons, a fellow of the American Orthopaedic Association, a fellow of the American College of Surgeons, and a member of the American Surgical Association. He received the Nicolas Andry Award, the highest honor of the Association of Bone and Joint Surgeons, and the Kappa Delta Ann Doner Vaughn Award from the American Academy of Orthopaedic Surgeons. Dr. Laurencin served as Dean of the Medical School and Vice President for Health Affairs at the University of Connecticut. Previous to that he served as the Lillian T. Pratt Distinguished Professor of Orthopaedic Surgery and Chair of the Department of Orthopaedic Surgery at the University of Virginia.

Dr. Laurencin is an elected member of the National Academy of Sciences, an elected member of the National Academy of Engineering, an elected member of the National Academy of Medicine, and an elected fellow of the National Academy of Inventors. He is the first surgeon in history elected to all four of the Dr. Laurencin's scientific work has been marked by rigor, ingenuity, creativity, and originality. He is internationally renowned for work in biomaterials, stem cell science, nanotechnology, and drug delivery systems. His most outstanding achievements have fallen into four areas: the study of composites of polymers and ceramics for bone regeneration, the development of polymeric nanofiber technology for tissue regeneration, the use of polymer fiber matrices for the regeneration of soft tissue of the knee, and his new work in regenerative engineering.

This is Dr. Laurencin's Science

Polymer−ceramic systems

Dr. Laurencin pioneered the development of polymer−ceramic systems for bone regeneration. He created emulsion systems that resulted in sintered polymeric matrices for bone regeneration, and later combined them with low crystalline hydroxyapatite materials to create polymer−ceramic composites for bone regeneration. His seminal papers and patents have been the basis for an entire industry that utilizes polymer−ceramics for such devices as interference screws and engineered bone grafts. As a consultant to the major orthopaedic companies such as Stryker, and Smith and Nephew companies, Dr. Laurencin inspired the development of these implants. The biocomposite interference screw is a principal means of bone to soft tissue fixation in anterior cruciate ligament reconstruction. Dr. Laurencin's work, in publications and patents, has served as an important basis for the field (over 500,000 ACL reconstructions are performed worldwide and at least 25% of these utilize biocomposite screws). In the area of bone grafts for repair, Dr. Laurencin's basic and translational work inspired the development of the Microfuse bone repair system based on polymer and polymer/ceramic materials. Developed by Globus Medical, Inc., Dr. Laurencin currently receives royalties from the product. To our knowledge, this is one of the few engineered materials inspired products finding widespread use on the clinical market.

In his latest work in the field, he has combined polymer−ceramic systems with nanofiber technology to create unique inductive matrices for bone regeneration. (See Nelson, C., Khan YM, and Laurencin CT: Nanofiber−microsphere (nano−micro) matrices for bone regenerative engineering: a convergence approach toward matrix design. Regenerative Biomaterials 1, 3−9 (2014) (Lead Article for the Journal). The work has resulted in the ability to create matrices that induce bone without the use of morphogenetic proteins. At the same time, Dr. Laurencin has worked to explore the use of graphene for bone regeneration using his sintering technology. Through unique graphene oxide chemistry, calcium phosphate ceramic is created, and through controlled delivery of calcium, an inductive, high strength matrix is formed. Using a transgenic mouse model, the ability of these systems to differentiate stem cells to bone was found. This work has been published in the Proceedings of the National Academy of Sciences with Dr. Laurencin as cocorresponding author (Arnold, A, Holt, B, Daneshmandi, L, Laurencin, CT, Sydlik, SA. Phosphate graphene as an intrinsically osteoinductive scaffold for stem cell-driven bone regeneration. *Proc Natl Acad Sci.* 2019 Feb 22. https://doi.org/10.1073/pnas. 1815434116).

It should be noted that Dr. Laurencin was named one of the 100 Engineers of the Modern Era by the American Institute of Chemical Engineers at its Centennial Celebration. He was named specifically for his trailblazing work in the development of polymer−ceramics systems for bone regeneration. More recently, Dr. Laurencin has been elected a fellow in Polymeric Materials

Science and Engineering by the PMSE section of the American Chemical Society. He received the Kappa Delta Award (highest honor) from the American Association of Orthopaedic Surgeons for his work entitled "30 Years of Bone Regenerative Engineering."

Polymeric Nanofibers for Tissue Regeneration

Dr. Laurencin is regarded as the individual who heralded the use of nanotechnology for tissue regeneration and engineering. Regarding polymeric nanofibers, his breakthrough achievement described in early papers and seminal patents in the field (e.g., Laurencin, CT, Ko, FK. *Hybrid nanofibril matrices for use as tissue engineering devices.* US Patent No. 6,689,166) set the stage for the launch of an entire field. The nanofiber technology work has not only created new knowledge and technologies that have crossed over to medicine and biomedical engineering but also launched new fields outside of medicine. For instance, Jian Yong Feng, Jian Chun Zhang, Daxiang Yang in "Preparation and Oil Filtration Properties of Electrospun Nanofiber Composite Material" in the *Journal of Engineered Fibers and Fabrics*, Volume 9, Issue 4—2014, directly cite Laurencin and his group in describing the history of their adaptation of his technology for nonbiological purposes. His paper was selected for the cover of the special 100th volume anniversary edition of the *Journal of Biomedical Materials Research* detailing the top 25 papers of the past 50 years. Polymeric nanofiber technologies form the basis of much research today, and Laurencin's seminal patent (with Dr. Frank Ko) and seminal papers represent the start of the polymeric nanofiber field in biomedical engineering research.

His most recent work has involved the design and study of unique three-dimensional systems for tissue regeneration using nanofibers (Laurencin, CT, McLaughlin, SW, Veronick, J, Kahn, Y, Nair, LS, Goldhamer, DJ. *Bi-phasic 3-Dimensional Nanofiber Scaffolds, Two Parallel Beam Collector Device and Methods of Use.* US Patent No. 10,179,039) and the use of nanofiber technology to create artificial stem cell niches to control stem cell paracrine function (Peach, SM, Ramos, DM, James, R, Morozowich, N, Mazzocca, A, Doty, SB, Allcock, H, Kumbar, S, Laurencin, C. Engineered stem cell niche matrices for rotator cuff tendon regenerative engineering. *PLoS One.* 2017;12:e0174789. https://doi.org/10.1371/journal.pone.0174789). His work has explored muscle regeneration through the development of unique electroconductive matrices that preserve muscle function while stimulating regeneration (Tang X, Khan Y, Laurencin CT. Electroconductive nanofiber scaffolds for muscle regenerative engineering. *Front. Bioeng. Biotechnol.* 2017;8(x):8—12. https://doi.org/10.3389/conf.FBIOE.2016.01.02165).

The Regeneration of Soft Tissues of the Knee

Dr. Laurencin's studies have taken us from a basic understanding of soft tissue/material interaction events through to preclinical testing of matrices for soft tissue regeneration, through to clinical trials. He challenged the long-held dogma that regeneration of musculoskeletal tissues necessitated the use of morphogenetic factors to take place. His research over a period of 15 years resulted in the development of the Laurencin—Cooper (LC) ligament for anterior cruciate ligament regeneration (knee) and the STR graft for rotator cuff regeneration (shoulder). The shoulder rotator cuff regeneration product has been cleared for use by the FDA, and the anterior cruciate ligament device has now been implanted in humans as part of a large clinical trial in Europe. It should be noted that the development of the LC ligament was highlighted by National Geographic Magazine in its "100 Discoveries that Changed the World" edition. The work performed in the development of the LC ligament demonstrates his ability to move from the highly basic science level of research to applied materials research and finally to clinical applications. It has been through the unique intersection of his background that he has asked important questions in an interdisciplinary way that has resulted in the forging of new science, new technologies, and new solutions in biomedical engineering.

Dr. Laurencin's new work has built upon understanding the basic regenerative processes governing soft tissue of the knee, and exploring and developing next generation technologies. Most recently, he has explored bone—soft tissue interface regeneration in engineered ligament systems (Mengsteab PY, Conroy P, Badon M, Otsuka T, Kan H-M, Vella AT, Nair LS, Laurencin CT. Evaluation of a bioengineered ACL matrix's osteointegration with BMP-2 supplementation. *PLoS One*. 2020;15(1):e0227181. https://doi.org/10.1371/journal.pone.0227181), the design of high strength graft systems for regeneration (Laurencin, CT, Nair, LS, Mengsteab, PY, Kan, HM. *Bioengineered Double ACL Matrix*. US Patent Application 63/010,102), and studies on enhanced ACL regeneration through the use of stem cells (Yu, X, Mengsteab, PY, Narayanan, G, Nair, LS, Laurencin, CT. Enhancing the surface properties of a bioengineered anterior cruciate ligament matrix for use with point-of-care stem cell therapy, *Engineering*. 2020. https://doi.org/10.1016/j.eng.2020.02.010).

The totality of his work in tissue regeneration earned him the National Medal of Technology and Innovation, our nation's highest honor for technological achievement, awarded by the President of the United States.

Regenerative Engineering

Laurencin's new work has taken on bold, novel directions. He believes that a convergence approach to regeneration, using disparate technologies from such areas as nanotechnology and developmental biology, hold the key for accomplishing complex tissue regeneration. He has termed this new field "regenerative engineering." Convergence is an approach to problem solving that cuts across disciplinary boundaries. It integrates knowledge, tools, and ways of thinking from life and health sciences, physical, mathematical, and computational sciences, engineering disciplines, and beyond to form a comprehensive synthetic framework for tackling scientific and societal challenges that exist at the interfaces of multiple fields. By merging these diverse areas of expertise in a network of partnerships, convergence stimulates innovation from basic science discovery to translational application. It provides fertile ground for new collaborations that engage stakeholders and partners not only from academia but also from national laboratories, industry, clinical settings, and funding bodies. Knowledge created by the process of convergence can contribute to understanding complex biological systems while fostering medically relevant solutions, and this is Dr. Laurencin's main focus today.

Dr. Laurencin's work in regenerative engineering has resulted in a textbook in the field, and he is editor-in-chief of *Regenerative Engineering and Translational Medicine*, published by Springer Nature. He is the founder and president of the Regenerative Engineering Society, now a community within the American Institute of Chemical Engineers. The new society is highly collaborative. Meetings are often held in conjunction with other societies. For instance, this year the Regenerative Engineering Society had its combined meeting with the Society for Biomaterials. In education, the University of Connecticut Board of Trustees approved the first master's degree program in Regenerative Engineering. Most recently, Dr. Laurencin became the principal investigator for NIH's first predoctoral training grant (NIH T32) in regenerative engineering.

Dr. Laurencin's new research work has brought insights in stem cell science and developmental biology into traditional areas of biomedical engineering research in finding new ways to medically engineer tissues. For instance, his studies on stem cells (Zhibo, S, Nair, LS, Laurencin, CT. The paracrine effect of adipose-derived stem cells inhibits IL-1B-induced inflammation in chondrogenic cells through the WNT-B catenin signaling pathway. *Regen. Eng. Transl. Med.* 2018;4:35−41) have described pathways by which adipose-derived stem cells regenerate cartilage, while his work in salamanders has found a discrete group of cells that are responsible for limb regeneration (Otsuka T, Phan A, Laurencin, CT, Esko JD, Bryant SV and Gardiner DM. Identification of Heparan-Sulfate Rich Cells in the Loose Connective Tissues of the Axolotl (*Ambystoma mexicanum*) with the Potential to Mediate Growth Factor Signaling during Regeneration. *Regen. Eng. Transl. Med.* 2020. https://doi.org/10.1007/s40883-019-00140-3). Remarkably, he has found that these heparan sulfate-rich cells are also found in mammalian tissue, forging a new line of research and discovery in the quest for limb regeneration.

More About Dr. Laurencin

Dr. Laurencin is the pioneer of the new field, regenerative engineering. He is an expert in biomaterials science, stem cell technology, and nanotechnology and was named one of the 100 Engineers of the Modern Era by the American Institute of Chemical Engineers. He received the Founder's Award (highest award) from the Society for Biomaterials, the Von Hippel Award (highest award) from the Materials Research Society, and the James Bailey Award (highest award) from the Society for Biological Engineering. He received the NIH Director's Pioneer Award, NIH's highest and most prestigious research award, for his new field of regenerative engineering and the National Science Foundation's Emerging Frontiers in Research and Innovation Grant Award. Dr. Laurencin is the editor-in-chief of *Regenerative Engineering and Translational Medicine*, published by Springer Nature, and is the founder of the Regenerative Engineering Society. He is a fellow of the American Chemical Society, a fellow of the American Institute for Medical and Biological Engineering, a fellow of the American Institute of Chemical Engineers, a fellow of the Biomedical Engineering Society, a Fellow of the American Ceramic Society, a fellow of the Materials Research Society, an international fellow in Biomaterials Science and Engineering, and an international fellow in Medical and Biological Engineering. The American Association for the Advancement of Science awarded Dr. Laurencin the Philip Hauge Abelson Prize given "for signal contributions to the advancement of science in the United States."

Dr. Laurencin is active in mentoring, especially underrepresented minority students. He received the American Association for the Advancement of Science (AAAS) Mentor Award, the Beckman Award for Mentoring, and the Presidential Award for Excellence in Science, Math and Engineering Mentoring in ceremonies at the White House. These are the three principal national awards for mentoring. The Society for Biomaterials established the Cato T. Laurencin, MD, PhD Travel Fellowship in his honor, awarded to underrepresented minority students pursuing research. Dr. Laurencin is also active in addressing Health Disparities. Dr. Laurencin completed the Program in African-American Studies at Princeton University. He is a core faculty member of the Africana Studies Institute at the University of Connecticut and is editor-in-chief of the *Journal of Racial and Ethnic Health Disparities*, published by Springer Nature. He cofounded the W. Montague Cobb/NMA Health Institute, dedicated to addressing Health Disparities, and served as its founding chair. The W. Montague Cobb/NMA Health Institute and the National Medical Association established the Cato T. Laurencin Lifetime Research Achievement Award, given during the opening ceremonies of the National Medical Association Meeting.

At the National Academies, he is the founding chair of the National Academies Roundtable on Black Men and Black Women in Science, Engineering and Medicine. Dr. Laurencin conceived of the idea and raised funds from foundations to begin the initiative. The Roundtable has been highly impactful, and its website is https://www.nationalacademies.org/our-work/roundtable-on-black-men-and-black-women-in-science-engineering-and-medicine. Honored for his contribution to Black racial social justice and equity, Dr. Laurencin has been named a 2020 Healthcare Hero by Connecticut Magazine where he addressed how and why COVID-19 is disproportionately affecting the Black Community. Dr. Laurencin accepted the Herbert W. Nickens Award from the American Association of Medical Colleges "for his monumental contributions to promoting justice in medical education and health care equity throughout the nation." During Dr. Laurencin's remarks, he outlined what he termed the "IDEAL Pathway" to achieving and equitable and just society. The video can be found here: https://health.uconn.edu/connecticut-convergence-institute/2020/11/23/ideal-pathway-video/.

Dr. Laurencin is an elected fellow of the American Academy of Arts and Sciences and an elected fellow of the American Association for the Advancement of Science. Active internationally, he is an elected fellow of the Indian National Academy of Sciences, the Indian National Academy of Engineering, the African Academy of Sciences, and the World Academy of Sciences and is an academician of the Chinese Academy of Engineering. Dr. Laurencin is a fellow of the Royal Academy of Engineering.

Dr. Laurencin is a recipient of the Hoover Medal. Established in 1929, this medal commemorates the civic and humanitarian achievements of engineers. It is conferred upon an engineer whose professional achievements and personal endeavors have advanced the well-being of humankind. It is given jointly by five societies: the American Society of Mechanical Engineers, the American Society of Civil Engineers, the American Institute of Chemical Engineers, the American Institute of Mining, Metallurgical and Petroleum Engineers, and the Institute of Electrical and Electronics Engineers.

Dr. Laurencin is the 106th recipient of the Spingarn Medal. It is the highest honor of the NAACP given "to the man or woman of African descent and American citizenship who shall have made the highest achievement during the preceding year or years in any honorable field." He is the recipient of the UNESCO Equatorial Guinea International Prize for Research in the Life Sciences bestowed in ceremonies at the meeting of the African Union in Ethiopia.

Dr. Laurencin is the recipient of the National Medal of Technology and Innovation, America's highest honor for technological achievement, awarded by President Barack Obama in ceremonies at the White House. He is the first individual in history to receive the oldest/highest award of the National Academy of Medicine (the Walsh McDermott Medal) and the oldest/highest award of the National Academy of Engineering (the Simon Ramo Founder's Award).

Chapter 4

Dr. Cato T. Laurencin 2022

In various parts of this book, I have talked about important aspects of my work, and the recognition that I have received. I thought it would be good to provide a summary of where I am in 2022. I hope this summary will be particularly useful for young people. I encourage them to dream big, use the lessons I have provided in this book, and never let anyone hold them back.

I was born and raised in the inner city of North Philadelphia. I am an alumnus of Central High School. I then earned a BSE in chemical engineering from Princeton University. I earned an MD, Magna Cum Laude, from the Harvard Medical School, and received the Robinson Award for Surgery. Simultaneously I earned my PhD in Biochemical Engineering/Biotechnology from MIT where I was named a Hugh Hampton Young Fellow.

I am an American engineer, physician, scientist, innovator, and a University Professor of the University of Connecticut. And as you have read in the other sections of this book, I am the Chief Executive Officer of the Connecticut

Convergence Institute for Translation in Regenerative Engineering.

I am proud to be regarded as the founder of the field of regenerative engineering, and am the editor-in-chief of the journal, *Regenerative Engineering and Translational Medicine*, and I am the founder and president of the Regenerative Engineering Society. The American Institute of Chemical Engineers created the Cato T. Laurencin Regenerative Engineering Founder's Award in recognition of my pioneering the field. In engineering and medicine, I am an elected member of the National Academy of Engineering, an elected member of the National Academy of Medicine, and an elected member of the National Academy of Sciences. I am the first individual in history to receive both the oldest/highest award from the National Academy of Engineering (the Simon Ramo Founder's Award) and one of the oldest/highest awards of the National Academy of Medicine (the Walsh McDermott Medal). I am the first surgeon in history to be elected to all four national academies (including the National Academy of Inventors) of the United States.

Success Is What You Leave Behind. https://doi.org/10.1016/B978-0-12-417224-1.00005-5

In science, I received the Philip Hauge Abelson Prize, from the American Association for the Advancement of Science, for "signal contributions to the advancement of science in the United States" for work in regenerative engineering.

In innovation, I was awarded the National Medal of Technology and Innovation, America's highest honor for technological advancement, awarded by President Barack Obama in ceremonies at the White House.

My Contributions to Engineering and Medicine

I have worked hard over decades in this field and am seen as a world leader in biomaterials, polymeric materials science, nanotechnology, stem cell science, and drug delivery systems. Papers and patents are key to this kind of work, and I have over 500, many that have had broad impact on human health, including launching the use of polymeric nanotechnology in musculoskeletal regeneration and ushering in a new era in orthopaedic therapies. My colleagues and I were the first to develop nanofiber technologies for tissue regeneration. In addition, I pioneered the development of polymer—ceramic systems for bone regeneration and inspired technologies on the market for bone repair/regeneration and for bioceramic implants such as interference screws for musculoskeletal repair.

I have worked in the development of systems for soft tissue regeneration and also invented the Laurencin—Cooper ligament (LC ligament) for ACL regeneration, and engineered grafts for shoulder rotator cuff tendon repair and regeneration. National Geographic highlighted the LC ligament in its "100 Scientific Discoveries that Changed the World" edition in 2012.

My Work in Chemical Engineering

I am a professor of Chemical and Biomolecular Engineering at the University of Connecticut. I was named one of the 100 Engineers of the Modern Era by the American Institute of Chemical Engineers for my work in pioneering polymer—ceramic systems for musculoskeletal use. As a fellow of the American Institute of Chemical Engineers, I won the William Grimes Award from the American Institute of Chemical Engineers, and I served on the Board of Directors of the American Institute of Chemical Engineers with a term from 2018 to 2021.

I am the founder and president of the Regenerative Engineering Society, a community within the American Institute of Chemical Engineers, and am the editor-in-chief of *Regenerative Engineering and Translational Medicine*, published by *Springer/Nature*. I am also the recipient of the James Bailey Award of the American Institute of Chemical Engineers and received the Percy Julian Medal, the highest award of the National Organization of Black Chemists and Chemical Engineers, and a fellow of the American Chemical Society.

Obtaining the recognition through awards has been gratifying. But understanding the people behind the names is important. Therefore, I want to provide a bit of a drill down on some of the awards.

In 2020, I was the recipient of the James E. Bailey award in Biological Engineering. The award is sponsored by the Society of Biological Engineering and is presented to an individual who is a pioneer, a mentor, an innovator, an integrator of biology and engineering, and a teacher, and whose achievements have provided a major impact to the field of biological engineering. In addition to receiving the prestigious award, I provided the James E. Bailey lecture titled *Regenerative Engineering: The Present and Future of Tissue Regeneration.*

James Edward Bailey, better known as Jay Bailey, was an international leader in the area of biochemical engineering. He was known as the most influential biochemical engineer of the modern times. He was lauded as having great ingenuity and creativity, and was characterized as an innovator. He himself was the recipient of the first Merck Award in Metabolic Engineering. He died too young, but his legacy lives on.

Percy Lavon Julian is one of my scientific heroes. He was a research chemist that pioneered the chemical synthesis of medicinal drugs from plants. He did so at great odds. He was born in the segregated south, but with utter determination, he was able to train in chemistry at the highest levels. In 2014, I won the 2014 Percy L. Julian Award for significant contributions in pure and/or applied research in science or engineering. Dr. Julian obtained his BS in Chemistry from DePauw University in 1920. Although he entered DePauw as a "substandard freshman," he graduated as the class valedictorian with Phi Beta Kappa honors. His first job was as an instructor at Fisk University. Julian left Fisk and obtained a master's degree in chemistry from Harvard in 1928 and his PhD in 1931 from the University of Vienna, Austria. It was after his return to DePauw in 1933 that Julian conducted the research that led to the synthesis of physostigmine, a drug used in the treatment of glaucoma. Julian left DePauw in 1936 to become director of research of the Soya Products Division of the Glidden Company in Chicago. This position at Glidden made Julian the world's first African American to lead a research group in a major corporation. Dr. Julian rewarded Glidden's faith in him by producing many new commercial products from soybeans.

As an entrepreneur as well as a scientist, in 1953, he founded Julian Laboratories and later Julian Associates, Inc., and the Julian Research Institute. Over the course of his career, he acquired over 130 patents, including one for a fire-extinguishing foam that was used on oil and gasoline fires during World War II. Though he had over 130 patents and 200 scientific publications, his most notable contribution was in the synthesis of steroids from soy and sweet potato products. His founding his own company and pioneering the industrial large-scale syntheses of a number of human hormones was truly remarkable. He was in effect responsible for the development of an entire industry involving steroid hormones. Percy Julian was the inventor on over 130 patents. When he had difficulty translating his patents to licensing dollars, he invented his own company that made the intermediates for chemical syntheses. Julian and his team (with many Black scientists) successfully synthesized intermediates to such a fine extent that companies came to him to purchase them. Percy Julian was the first Black chemist inducted into the National Academy of Sciences. When I was elected to the National Academy of Sciences, I was elected in the engineering sciences section. But, in honor of Percy Julian, I designated my secondary section as Chemistry. His spirit and his legacy live on.

My Work in Materials Science and Engineering

In addition, I am a professor of Materials Science and Engineering at the University of Connecticut. In Materials Science and Engineering, I am a fellow of the Materials Research Society and have been the Fred Kavli Distinguished Lecturer and Plenary Speaker for the Materials Research Society. I am a life member of the American Ceramic Society and have delivered two of their most prestigious lectures. I have served as the Edward Orton, Jr., Memorial Lecturer and the Rustum Roy Lecturer for the American Ceramic Society. I am a fellow of the American Ceramics Society (ACers) and have been named one of the most highly cited researchers in Material Science and Engineering (Scopus). As an expert in polymers, I am a fellow of the American Chemical Society, and also a fellow in Polymeric Science and Engineering (PMSE) in the American Chemical Society.

I received the highest award of the Materials Research Society, the Von Hippel Award. Again, the specialness of some awards is in their background and in their specific meaning. The Von Hippel Award is the Materials Research Society's highest honor, and it "recognizes those qualities most prized by materials scientists and engineers—brilliance and originality of intellect, combined with vision that transcends the boundaries of conventional scientific disciplines." In receiving the award, I had the opportunity to delve into the background of Dr. Arthur Von Hippel. Fortunately, Dr. Mildred Dresselhaus, a very famous professor at MIT, published a paper entitled "Arthur Von Hippel: the Man Behind the Von Hippel Award." I believe I had much in common with Von Hippel. First I learned that he was on the faculty at MIT. He in fact had been at MIT during the time I completed my PhD at MIT and also, when I was on the faculty of the school. Second, he was someone that embraced a number of scientific disciplines in his work. Third, he was socially conscious. He supported and encouraged women to gain training in Materials Science at MIT. I am proud to have received the Von Hippel Award and proud to be among the ranks of those associated with his name.

My Work in Biomedical Engineering

I am also a professor of Biomedical Engineering. My work has been honored at the White House, receiving the Presidential Faculty Fellow Award from President Bill Clinton for my efforts merging engineering and medicine. And I am a fellow of the International Academy of Medical and Biological Engineering. In addition, I am an international fellow in Biomaterials Science and Engineering, a fellow of the American Institute for Medical and Biomedical Engineering, and a fellow of the Biomedical Engineering Society. My work was honored by Scientific American magazine as one of the "50 Greatest Achievements in Science" in 2007.

More recently, I received the Act Biomaterialia Gold Medal. Besides being recognized with an honor bestowed to others who I highly respect, it is the meaning behind the award that is important to me. The award is given for biomaterials research "that has had a significant and lasting impact on the development of the discipline, or recent work of great originality." The selection of the individual is based as follows: "The awardee should be a recognized world leader in the field of biomaterials, whose accomplishments in discovery and translation to practice are surpassing and well known in the field." The committee awarding the medal represent some of the most accomplished individuals in the biomaterials field. I am especially grateful to them for recognizing the quality of my work and my vision.

I am active in technology development. My philosophy has always been that engineering is the bridge between science and society. Those engaged in engineering research have an obligation to translate research discoveries to the benefit of people. In 2012, my work in musculoskeletal tissue regeneration was featured in National Geographic magazine's "100 Discoveries that Changed Our World" edition.

In addition, I received the Technology, Innovation and Development Award from the Society for Biomaterials in 2013 for key scientific and technical innovation and leadership in translational research. In Connecticut, I was named Academic Entrepreneur of the Year by Connecticut Cure for my work in technology development, and I have received the Connecticut Medal of Technology and Innovation.

In 2009, I won the Pierre Galletti Award, medical and biological engineering's greatest honor. I felt a great deal of kinship with Dr. Pierre Galletti even though I did not know him well. Dr. Pierre M. Galletti was a leading researcher on artificial organs and tissue engineering. He wrote very clear monographs on these subjects and influenced my decision to become an engineer, even when I was in high school. He died from a fall at home. To this day, I work to keep my home as safe as possible for myself and for my family. I think of where our science of tissue regeneration could be now, if he were alive.

Dr. Galletti worked in using cells combined with polymeric matrices for use in engineering tissues. He worked in the cardiovascular area in his research, while my work focused on the creation of matrices in the musculoskeletal arena. Galletti became a professor at Brown in 1967. I was only seven at the time. He served for almost 20 years as Vice President of the Biology and Medicine Division at Brown. Like most gifted scientist/engineers, he worked to translate his technologies to help people. In 1988, he was one the founding scientists of Cellular Transplants Inc., a biotechnology company that became Cytotherapeutics Inc. He was the editor-in-chief of the journal *Cardiology* and the editor in chief of *The Journal of the American Society for Artificial Internal Organs* from 1978 to 1985. The latter journal was extremely prominent in the field during the time of graduate study at MIT. Thus, Pierre Galletti had a lasting influence on me from secondary school, to graduate school, to my entering faculty positions.

My Work in Medicine

I am the Albert and Wilda Van Dusen Distinguished Endowed Professor of Orthopaedic Surgery at the University of Connecticut. I completed residency training at the Harvard Combined Orthopaedic Surgery Program, where I was chief resident in Orthopaedic Surgery at the Beth Israel Hospital, Harvard Medical School. I served as vice president for Health Affairs and dean of the School of Medicine at the University of Connecticut. Previous to that, I served as the Lillian T. Pratt Distinguished Professor of Orthopaedic Surgery and Orthopaedic Surgeon-In-Chief at the University of Virginia Health System.

While I am a researcher and scientist, I am also a board-certified shoulder and knee surgeon. I am proud to have been named to America's Top Doctors (15th consecutive year) from Castle Connolly and I have been named to "America's Leading Physicians" by Black Enterprise magazine. I have also been named to Connecticut's Top Doctors.

I have had the opportunity to serve as a ringside boxing physician (which is a long story, and perhaps for another book) and have been a physician for the USA Boxing men's elite team. I have been a member of the USA Boxing National Medical Advisory Board. I am also a fellow of the American Academy of Orthopaedic Surgeons, a fellow of the American Orthopaedic Association, a fellow of the American College of Surgeons, and an elected member of the American Surgical Association. I received the Nicolas Andry Award, the highest honor of the Association of Bone and Joint Surgeons. I also received the Kappa Delta Award, one of the highest awards of the American Academy of Orthopaedic Surgeons. As of this date (2022), I am currently the only living orthopaedic surgeon elected to the American Academy of Arts and Sciences. I also have received an honorary degree from the Mount Sinai School of Medicine in 2018.

I also received the 2019 UNESCO-Equatorial Guinea International Prize for Research in the Life Sciences, becoming the first American to earn this prestigious award. The ceremony took place during the Africa Union Heads of States Summit located in Addis Ababa, Ethiopia, in 2020.

The Prize is awarded to a maximum of three laureates who have made significant efforts through scientific research toward improving the quality of human life. I had the privilege of being formally selected by the UNESCO Director-General for my fundamental contributions in the field of regenerative engineering, the field I pioneered. In receiving the award, I was recognized worldwide as a leader in biomaterials, nanotechnology, stem cell science, drug delivery systems, and regenerative engineering.

I was humbled and invigorated to receive the only International Prize in Science given by the continent of Africa. As the first person from the African Diaspora to receive this award, it in a way rededicated me to expanding the field of regenerative engineering, to create new solutions for the world.

My Work in Equity and Justice

In addition to my career in science and medicine, I am deeply passionate about creating opportunities for, and mentoring of underrepresented Black, Indigenous, and People of Color. I received the American Association for the Advancement of Science (AAAS) Mentor Award, the Beckman Award for Mentoring, and the Presidential Award for Excellence in Science, Math and Engineering Mentoring in ceremonies at the White House. The Society for Biomaterials established the Cato T. Laurencin, MD, PhD, Travel Fellowship in his honor, given to underrepresented students pursuing research. I am proud to have received an honorary degree from Lincoln University, one of the oldest historically Black colleges in the country.

All of the mentor awards have been special. Established by the AAAS Board of Directors in 1996, the Mentor Award honors AAAS members who have mentored significant numbers of underrepresented students (women, minorities, and persons with disabilities) toward a PhD degree in the sciences, as well as scholarship, activism, and community-building on behalf of underrepresented groups in science, technology, engineering, and mathematics fields.

Throughout my career, I have taken significant steps to ensure that the impact of his pioneering work in biomaterials and tissue engineering benefits both the research community and, through mentoring, future scientists and engineers. "His track record as an advocate for and a mentor to underrepresented minority students, teachers, and faculty is exemplary," said Yolanda S. George, deputy director of Education and Human Resources at AAAS. "Over the past 22 years, more than 90 underrepresented minority students at the undergraduate, graduate, and postgraduate levels have undertaken research projects in his various institutional laboratories," George added. "Considering that only a handful of African Americans hold tenure-track appointments in biomedical engineering nationally," George said, "it is difficult to overstate the impact that Dr. Laurencin has had on diversity in this field."

When I received the AAAS Mentor Award, my citation was "for his transformative impact and scientific contributions toward mentoring students in the field of biomedical engineering." It was at the awards ceremony that stated my vision for writing a book that would be lessons and tools for success in the world.

President Barack Obama honored me and 21 other recipients with the Presidential Award for Excellence in Science, Mathematics and Engineering Mentoring at the White House. It was to be the first of two honors I would receive from President Obama.

"We are here today to honor teachers and mentors who are upholding their responsibility not just to the young people who they teach but to our country by inspiring and educating a new generation in math and science," President Obama said. "But we're also here because this responsibility can't be theirs alone. All of us have a role to play in building an education system that is worthy of our children and ready to help us seize the opportunities and meet the challenges of the 21st century."

President Obama told the award recipients, "Whether it's showing students how to record the habits of a resident reptile, or teaching kids to test soil samples on a class trip to Costa Rica; whether it's helping young people from tough neighborhoods in Chicago to become 'Junior Paleontologists,' or creating a mentoring program that connects engineering students with girls and minorities, who are traditionally underserved in the field—all of you are demonstrating why teaching and mentoring is so important, and why we have to support you, equip you, and send in some reinforcements for you."

I am still humbled and honored by this award. Mentoring aspiring physicians, scientists, and engineers has been, and continues to be, one of the most gratifying aspects of my career.

I have been happy to help support young physicians, scientists, and researchers through specific programming. I believe these programs can become models for other institutions to use throughout the country.

Young Innovative Investigator Program

Our Young Innovative Investigator Program (YIIP) program aims to develop the next generation of innovative scientists by providing academic training to individuals dedicated to pursuing careers as scientists and scholars in biological and biomedical science. The program is specifically focused on recruiting underrepresented students to contribute toward developing a sustainable pipeline to increase diversity among the pool of academic scientists. YIIP provides tools for scholars to conduct research, succeed in an academic environment, and become competitive candidates for medical school or graduate school. YIIP scholars acquire the expertise necessary to obtain a PhD or MD/PhD or MD.

Research Experience Mentoring Program

Our Research Experience and Mentoring (REM) program aims to mentor students from diverse backgrounds to prepare them for careers in STEM-related disciplines. The program recruits high school students, undergraduate students, and teachers in professional development to provide them with skills including communications, scientific writing, and collaboration, while providing a high-quality research experience. Each summer, participants in the REM program are welcomed at UConn Health for research training. Participants learn the basic aspects of research including research problem identification, experimental design, and execution. Our laboratories have researchers at all levels (postdocs, grad students, undergraduate, and faculty members) so there is an opportunity to learn from a variety of scientists.

Presidential M1 Mentorship Award Program

In 2020, the Office of the Provost and the Connecticut Convergence Institute for Translation in Regenerative Engineering announced the selection of its 2020 Presidential M1 Mentorship Program Awardees. The four new M1 Mentors comprised a cadre of accomplished faculty members that aims to create a national model for best practices in mentorship of underrepresented racial and ethnic students and faculty in the biomedical sciences. Each M1 Mentor possesses high caliber mentoring experience, a commitment to engage and retain racial and ethnic underrepresented individuals along the biomedical science pipeline, and a record of success in securing research funding.

Building Infrastructure Leading to Diversity

The Building Infrastructure Leading to Diversity (BUILD) initiative provides awards to undergraduate institutions across the country to implement and study innovative approaches to engaging and retaining students from diverse backgrounds in biomedical research.

Doing the Work of Health Equity at the Community Level

It is important to support the pipeline of that next generation of Black and Brown physicians, engineers, and researchers. But it has been just as important to make sure that I make an impact on disparities on the ground, in communities.

One way I have been able to put that in motion is through the creation of Just Us Moving Project (JUMP), a program designed to improve diabetes control by reducing the hemoglobin A1C levels of people in African/Black and Hispanic/Latino American communities by encouraging increased physical activity. By promoting and tracking daily physical activities, we knew that the information learned in our study could help other African and Hispanic Americans who have diabetes. One of the core goals of JUMP, which is sponsored by the Aetna Foundation, is to educate the community on the importance of increased physical activity. Here at the Connecticut Convergence Institute, we believe that small changes in daily activity can result in substantial health benefits.

Another important part of my life has been my work as an expert in public health, especially as it pertains to ethnic minority health and health disparities. Academically, I completed the Program in African American Studies at Princeton University. I believe I was the first chemical engineering to complete such a program at Princeton. It was not clear how I would use the training in African American studies. I just used the lesson "If you do good things, good things happen." Fast forward to now, I am a core faculty member of the Africana Studies Institute at the University of Connecticut and is editor-in-chief of the *Journal of Racial and Ethnic Health Disparities*, published by *Springer/Nature*, a leading journal in the field. I have used my training to write landmark papers, including the first paper in the referred literature showing high levels of COVID-19 cases and deaths in Blacks. I currently serve as chair of the National Academies Roundtable on Black Men and Black Women in Science, Engineering, and Medicine.

Seeing a need to directly address issues facing Black people in health, I cofounded the W. Montague Cobb/NMA Health Institute, dedicated to addressing racial health disparities, and served as its first chair of the Board. I received excellent training and experience serving on the board of trustees of the National Medical Association for over a decade and was speaker of the House of Delegates of the National Medical Association. I am proud that the W. Montague Cobb/NMA Health Institute and the National Medical Association created the Cato T. Laurencin Lifetime Achievement Award. It is bestowed at the opening ceremonies of the annual meeting of the National Medical Association. The recipients have included luminaries in science including Jane Cooke Wright (first Black women to conduct cancer trials) to Mae Jemison (first Black woman astronaut).

In 2020, during the COVID-19 pandemic, the Association of American Medical Colleges (AAMC) awarded me the Herbert W. Nickens Award. The award is bestowed on an individual who has made monumental contributions to promoting justice in medical education and healthcare equity throughout the nation. My work in social justice over the past 40 years is a natural extension of the teaching of my parents and role models who always emphasized fairness and respect.

As a young medical student, I met Dr. Nickens. He was a towering figure, who truly passed at a very young age. Dr. Herbert W. Nickens was the founding vice president of the AAMC Division of Community and Minority Programs, now Diversity Policy and Programs. In some ways, he was a maverick. He certainly was a trailblazer demonstrating passionate leadership in describing issues facing Black, Indigenous and People of Color entering medicine. I am honored to have received an award named after him.

Perhaps it is fitting that the last award and its significance that I will discuss is the Spingarn Medal, for it sums up all aspects of my life to date. In March of 2021, I received an email from the NAACP. It was innocuous and asked me to review a letter attached and get back to them. To my surprise and delight, I had been awarded the Spingarn Medal. The opening words of the letter are etched in my memory.

Dear Dr. Laurencin, It is an honor, as well as a pleasure, for me to inform you that you have been selected to receive the 106th NAACP Spingarn Medal for 2021. The Spingarn Award Committee took this action at its closed meeting on Thursday, February 17, 2021. As you may recall, the Spingarn Medal was instituted in 1914 and is presented annually, to the man or woman of African descent, who shall have made the highest achievement in any honorable field of endeavor during the preceding year or years. On behalf of the Spingarn Award Committee, I extend our heartiest congratulations on an honor which you do indeed richly deserve.

The Spingarn Medal is, to me, the most iconic award presented in America, if not the world. Medalists include Dr. Martin Luther King, Jr, Maya Angelou, Harry Belafonte, Julian Bond, Honorable Robert L. Carter, Honorable John Conyers, Misty Copeland, Ruby Dee, Mrs. Frankie Muse Freeman, Earl G. Graves, Sr, Dorothy I. Height, Lena Horne, The Hon. Nathaniel R. Jones, Quincy Jones, Vernon Jordan, Honorable John Lewis, Jessye Norman, Gordon Parks, Sidney Poitier, The Hon. Colin Powell, Percy E. Sutton, Cicely Tyson, the late Carl Rowan, Myrlie Evers-Williams, Governor L. Douglas Wilder, and Oprah Winfrey, to name a few.

I am the first engineer to receive the Spingarn Medal; I am also the fifth physician and the fourth scientist to receive the Spingarn Medal. In awarding me the medal, the following is the press release for the Spingarn Medal.

BALTIMORE—The NAACP has announced that Cato T. Laurencin, MD, PhD, Van Dusen Distinguished Endowed Professor at the University of Connecticut, will be awarded the prestigious Spingarn Medal during the NAACP's 112nd Annual Convention.

The award recognizes Dr. Laurencin's seminal and singular accomplishments in tissue regeneration, biomaterials science, nanotechnology, and regenerative engineering, a field he founded. His exceptional career has made him the foremost engineer—physician—scientist in the world. His breakthrough achievements have resulted in transformative advances in improving human life. His fundamental contributions to materials science and engineering include introducing nanotechnology into the biomaterials field for regeneration.

> *"Dr. Laurencin's contribution to furthering humanity's collective achievement in the field of science and engineering is extraordinary," said Derrick Johnson, president and CEO, NAACP. "As a pioneer of the new field, Regenerative Engineering, he is shaping the landscape of cell-based therapy, gene therapy, and immunomodulation. Named as one of the 100 Engineers of the Modern Era by the American Institute of Chemical Engineers, he has received countless awards for his transformative work. The NAACP is proud to present Dr. Laurencin with our highest recognition and join the chorus of those that realize what his work means globally."*

Why the Spingarn Matters to Me

I am so blessed and honored to receive this amazing recognition and join the historic ranks of my fellow Spingarn Medal honorees. The NAACP Spingarn award was established in 1914 by the late Joel E. Spingarn—then NAACP Chairman of the Board of Directors. It was given annually until his death in 1939. The medal is awarded for the highest or noblest achievement by a living African American during the preceding year or years in any honorable field. Previous Spingarn medal recipients include Mrs. Daisy Bates (Little Rock Nine), Myrlie Evers-Williams, Earl G. Graves Sr, W.E.B DuBois, George Washington Carver, Charles Drew, Jackie Robinson, Martin Luther King, Jr, Jesse L. Jackson, Maya Angelou, Oprah Winfrey, Cicely Tyson, Harry Belafonte, Sidney Poitier, Quincy Jones, and the Honorable Nathaniel Jones.

I am honored to be the first surgeon in history to be elected to all four national academies: the National Academy of Sciences, the National Academy of Engineering, the National Academy of Medicine, and the National Academy of Inventors.

Founded in 1909 in response to the ongoing violence against Black people around the country, the NAACP (National Association for the Advancement of Colored People) is the largest and most preeminent civil rights organization in the nation. The NAACP mission is to secure the political, educational, social, and economic equality of rights to eliminate race-based discrimination and ensure the health and well-being of all persons.

While the Spingarn Medal recognized my work in regenerative engineering, I believe the committee also recognized my commitment to achieving a world of fairness and justice for all. I am particularly gratified to be in the company of such scientists as George Washington Carver, Ernest Just, and Percy Julian (with whom I mentioned earlier), who have performed transformative research to the benefit of humankind.

Epilogue: A Bit of Closing Philosophy

I was once interviewed by a magazine where they asked me about my life to date, what I have achieved, and what I am most proud of. I provided the following answer and included some philosophy. I think it may be a good way to close this book.

> *"In truth, the proud moments are too numerous to count. I am blessed and highly favored. The moments surrounding my family (meeting and falling in love with my wife, and the birth of my children probably count as the best moments). Speaking of moments, I want to share some of my philosophy. There are actually three 'most important' dates of your life. They are the day you are born, the day you realize your purpose in life, and the day you are truly carrying out your life on purpose. For me, starting a new field, Regenerative Engineering, taking care of patients as a surgeon, working for social justice, mentoring the next generation, all while doing the most important thing: staying connected to my family, my values and my God, collectively represent my purpose. A life on purpose is where I am, which is the ultimate goal."*

Afterword by Philip Bailey
(Lead Singer, Earth, Wind & Fire)

A musician and a physician meet in a hotel in Europe. All the way around the world. You'd think we wouldn't have much in common. There is the love of music, of course. But there is also the thing that happens when people who are passionate about their respective professions, they can bond in appreciation of excellence.

There is a story that you read in this book of how Dr. Laurencin was in a hotel bar in Europe and struck up a conversation with some Black men who looked "familiar." My bandmates, and I, you may know us as Earth Wind and Fire, had no idea that the man we were chatting with was a world-renowned engineer, scientist, and inventor. And we had no idea at all that he was one of the best sports medicine and shoulder doctors out there until we were telling him about one of our band members who was up in his room, because he had dislocated his shoulder. What are the chances that this encounter was with someone who would be able to set the shoulder back in place, but also a man who was working on regenerating limbs? We didn't even know such a thing was possible. It occurs to me that we also both have healing in common. I use my voice.

Fast forward to September 10, 2001. We were scheduled to perform in Philadelphia at a major venue. I remembered my friend Dr. Laurencin and so invited him to come to the Earth, Wind and Fire concert, and come backstage to be reunited with the bandmates. It was a memorable night and a memorable backstage. Remember, the date was September 10, 2001. We were scheduled to go to New York to perform at our next gig. The next day we and the world were shocked by the World Trade Center attack. Of course, our gig was called off, and we were stationed in Philadelphia.

I spent a number of days with Dr. Laurencin. He opened his home to me, and I met his wonderful family. But perhaps most of all, I was able to experience the man that he is. He was caring, confident, wise, and above all giving. The experience being with him cemented our lifelong friendship, and my lifelong admiration for him.

Fast forward again, it was 2011. I received a call from Dr. Laurencin. He was Dean of the University of Connecticut School of Medicine and had nominated me and secured my election to receive an honorary degree at the UConn School of Medicine. I was honored to receive an honorary degree from the University of Connecticut, presented by Dr. Laurencin himself, in what was a full circle moment. He and I both understand the healing power of music.

Success Is What You Leave Behind. https://doi.org/10.1016/B978-0-12-417224-1.00007-9

When I read Dr. Laurencin's book, *Success Is What You Leave Behind*, I could not help but be both impressed and inspired by the insights he shares. We both understand what it is like to work hard to be at the top of our game and what it takes to stay there. Our work has taken each of us all over the world. We have each worked to exhibit excellence in our careers and to push the boundaries of what is possible.

There are so many people who are looking for inspiration in their own journeys to excellence in their professions and in striving to have a fully formed life. They are looking to live "a life on purpose" as Dr. Laurencin states. This inspirational book sets a path. This is a must read. It was for me, and it is for you.

Index

Note: 'Page numbers followed by "*f*" indicate figures and "*t*" indicate tables.'

Printed and bound by CPI Group (UK) Ltd, Croydon, CR0 4YY

08/06/2025

01896869-0013